Critical Care Focus

Critical Care Focus

2: Respiratory failure

EDITOR

DR HELEN F GALLEY

Lecturer in Anaesthesia and Intensive Care
University of Aberdeen

EDITORIAL BOARD

PROFESSOR NIGEL R WEBSTER

Professor of Anaesthesia and Intensive Care
University of Aberdeen

DR PAUL G P LAWLER

Clinical Director of Intensive Care
South Cleveland Hospital

DR NEIL SONI

Consultant in Anaesthesia and Intensive Care
Chelsea and Westminster Hospital

DR MERVYN SINGER

Reader in Intensive Care
University College Hospital, London

First published in 1999
by the BMJ Publishing Group, BMA House, Tavistock Square,
London WC1H 9JR

www.bmjbooks.com

British Library Cataloguing in Publication Data

A catalogue record for this book is available from the British Library

ISBN 0-7279-1466-9

The chapters in this book are based on talks given at the Intensive Care Society's
"State of the Art" Meeting, Olympia Conference Centre, London,
December 1998.

Typeset by Phoenix Photosetting, Chatham, Kent
Printed and bound by J W Arrowsmith Ltd

Contents

Contributors   vii

1 Respiratory physiology of positive pressure ventilation   1
  ANDREW B LUMB

2 Non-invasive respiratory support in the intensive care unit   19
  MASSIMO ANTONELLI

3 What's new in ventilator weaning?   26
  LAURENT BROCHARD

4 Positioning in acute lung injury and acute respiratory distress
  syndrome   31
  ANTONIO PESENTI

5 The early fibrotic response in acute lung injury and the role
  of steroids   37
  GEOFF BELLINGAN

6 Capillary stress failure and pulmonary damage   52
  JOHN B WEST

Contributors

Massimo Antonelli
University La Sapienza, Rome, Italy

Geoff Bellingan
MRC Clinical Scientist and Honorary Senior Lecturer in Intensive Care Medicine, University College London Hospitals, London, UK

Laurent Brochard
Henri Mondor Hospital, France

Andrew B Lumb
Consultant Anaesthetist, St James's University Hospital, Leeds Teaching Hospitals NHS Trust, Leeds, UK

Antonio Pesenti
Università degli Studi di Milano, Ospedale S. Gerado, Monza, Italy

John B West
Professor of Medicine and Physiology, University of California San Diego, La Jolla, California, USA

1: Respiratory physiology of positive pressure ventilation

ANDREW B LUMB

Introduction

The introduction of general anaesthesia in the 19th century was soon followed by the occasional use of artificial ventilation, to remedy the periods of apnoea which occurred when anaesthesia became too "deep".[1] It was not until 1928 that Guedel and Waters, using an intratracheal catheter, used artificial ventilation deliberately.[2] A further twenty years elapsed before the first report of harmful effects of intermittent positive pressure ventilation (IPPV),[3] and this report described only the now well-known cardiovascular effects.[4] Adverse effects on the respiratory system are much more subtle, and their elucidation has been both piecemeal and slow.

Intermittent positive pressure ventilation

Studying physiological changes during IPPV is difficult. Conscious patients receiving artificial ventilation invariably have severely abnormal lung function, whilst patients receiving general anaesthesia commonly have healthy lungs but are subject to the many changes in lung physiology associated with anaesthesia and muscle relaxation.[5,6] In addition, provision of IPPV requires an air-tight seal with the patient's airway, in the form of either a cuffed tube in the trachea or a tight-fitting face mask. Both of these systems are associated with adverse respiratory effects, particularly tracheal tubes, which bypass the upper airway and larynx, so abolishing the ability of the respiratory centre to control expiratory flow rate.[7] It is therefore almost impossible to study the effects of IPPV alone. When interpreting studies of physiology during IPPV, great care must be taken to adequately account for abnormalities of lung function, the method of airway maintenance and the anaesthetic or sedative agents used. A summary of the respiratory changes seen with IPPV and positive end-expiratory pressure (PEEP) during general anaesthesia are shown in Table 1.1.

1

Table 1.1 Influence of anaesthesia and ventilatory mode on common respiratory variables

Ventilatory pattern	Pulmonary circulation				Ventilation			Blood gas tensions		
	Cardiac output (l/min)	Shunt (%)	PAP mean (mmHg)	PCWP (mmHg)	VE (l/min)	Paw mean (cmH$_2$O)	V_D/V_T (%)	PaO$_2$ (kPa)	PaCO$_2$ (kPa)	P(A–a)O$_2$ (kPa)
Awake – spontaneous	6.1 (0.6)	1.6	17 (6)	12 (7)	6.1 (1.4)	0	30	10.5 (1.7)	4.6 (1.2)	3.7 (1.4)
Anaesthetised – spontaneous	5.0 (0.3)	6.2	16 (6)	11 (6)	5.4 (1.4)	0	35	17.6 (6.3)	5.6 (0.4)	13.4 (6.1)
Anaesthetised – IPPV	4.5 (0.2)	8.6	18 (7)	13 (7)	7.0 (1.3)	8.5 (0.5)	38	18.8 (2.7)	4.9 (0.4)	13.1 (3.0)
Anaesthetised – PEEP 13 cmH$_2$O	3.7 (0.3)	4.1	25 (10)	18 (10)	6.0 (0.8)	20.7 (2.7)	44	20.5 (2.1)	5.8 (0.6)	12.5 (2.4)

Data are reproduced with permission from Bindslev LG et al., *Acta Anaesthesiol Scand* 1981;**25**:360–71[8] and show mean (SEM) values from 10 subjects of mean age 51 years. Fractional inspired oxygen (FIO$_2$) was 0.21 when awake and 0.4 during anaesthesia. PAP, pulmonary artery pressure; PCWP, pulmonary capillary wedge pressure; Paw, airway pressure.

Distribution of ventilation

Regional ventilation is determined by the compliance and time constants (resistance) of alveoli in different areas of the lung. With spontaneous breathing there is preferential ventilation of dependent areas of the lung, an observation first made by West in 1962.[9] This is caused by the weight of the lung above compressing alveoli in dependent areas, reducing their compliance. Studies performed recently in microgravity conditions on Spacelab have indicated that this long accepted explanation is not the whole story, in that some inhomogeneity of regional ventilation persists even when weightless,[10] although an explanation for this observation is lacking. At 1g, in the upright position, ventilation at the lung apex is only about one-third that at the lung base.[9] In the supine position, which is normally adopted for artificial ventilation, the gravity-dependent regional differences persist, but are of much smaller magnitude.[11,12] Results from an early study are shown in Figure 1.1, where ventilation at the top of the lung was about two-thirds of that in the dependent areas.[11] A more recent study using positron emission tomography (PET) to measure regional alveolar ventilation in supine subjects[12] found values of approximately 1.0 ml/min per ml of lung tissue at the top of the lung and a corresponding value of 2.2 ml/min at the bottom (Figure 1.1).

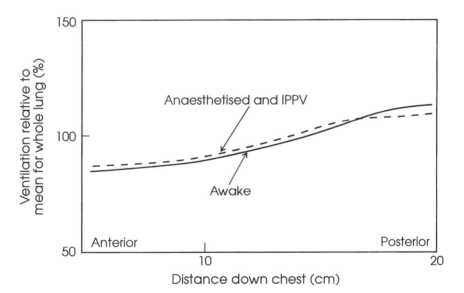

Figure 1.1   *Regional distribution of ventilation in horizontal slices of lung in healthy supine subjects. Both lines are derived from inspirations of 1 litre from functional residual capacity with normal flow rates. Note the almost identical distribution between awake spontaneous respiration and intermittent positive pressure ventilation (IPPV) during anaesthesia. Reproduced with permission from Hulands GH et al., Clin Sci 1970;38:451–60.[11]*

With IPPV, the same physiological factors determine the distribution of ventilation, and it may therefore be predicted that regional ventilation would be little different during IPPV compared with spontaneous breathing. The limited data available confirm this by showing only minor differences in regional ventilation during IPPV (Figure 1.2).

In diseased lungs, regional variations in compliance and resistance are substantial. Positive airway pressure, longer inspiratory times and variable inspiratory flow patterns may all then contribute to more homogeneous ventilation.[15] However, this may not necessarily be beneficial for gas exchange as perfusion of previously underventilated regions is also likely to be abnormal.

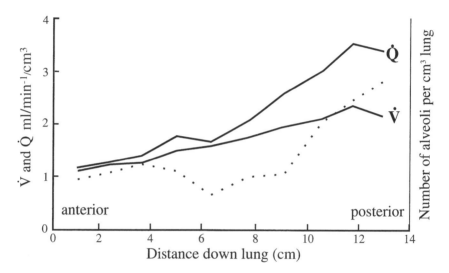

Figure 1.2   Vertical gradients in ventilation and perfusion in the supine position. Data are mean results from PET scans of 8 subjects during normal breathing, and for each vertical level represent the average value for a horizontal slice of lung. The solid lines relate to the left ordinate and are ventilation (V̇) and perfusion (Q̇) per ml of lung tissue. Ventilation and perfusion both increase on descending through the lung. The dotted line relates to the right ordinate and represents the number of alveoli per unit lung volume, which increases in dependent areas such that the blood flow per alveolus remains fairly constant. Derived from data in references 12 and 13, and reproduced with permission from Lumb AB. Nunn's applied respiratory physiology, 5th edn. Oxford: Butterworth-Heinemann, 2000.[14]

Distribution of perfusion

A positive pressure in the chest cavity is a significant physiological insult which under normal circumstances only occurs with coughing, straining, etc. Although these activities rarely last longer than a few seconds, the intrathoracic pressure achieved may be very high, for example, 120 cmH₂O during coughing. Artificial ventilation increases intrathoracic pressure by much more modest amounts, but these changes may be sustained for many hours or days. PEEP results in much larger increases in mean intrathoracic pressure than IPPV alone. For example, IPPV in a patient with normal lungs using 10 breaths of 10 ml/kg and an *I:E* ratio of 1:2 will generate mean airway pressures of approximately 5 cmH_2O. Addition of a modest 5 cmH_2O of PEEP will therefore double the mean airway pressure.

In normal lungs with spontaneous breathing, regional perfusion, like ventilation, is influenced by gravity with increased perfusion of dependent areas. Again, PET scanning in supine subjects has allowed precise quantification of regional perfusion, revealing values of 1.2 ml/min per ml of lung tissue in the upper lung, increasing to 3.5 ml/min in dependent areas (Figure 1.2).[12] This technique has also allowed quantification of alveolar size in different lung regions, and it can be seen from Figure 1.2 that the number of alveoli per ml of lung tissue increase in approximately the same way as the ventilation and perfusion. Thus perfusion *per alveolus* remains constant throughout the lung but the alveoli become smaller and so more numerous in dependent regions.

Pulmonary vascular resistance

An increase in intrathoracic pressure due to positive pressure ventilation will increase the pulmonary arterial intravascular pressure, which is normally measured relative to atmospheric pressure. There will also be a similar increase in pulmonary venous intravascular pressure and therefore driving pressure across the pulmonary vascular bed remains unchanged (Table 1.1). Thus when assessing pulmonary vascular resistance (PVR) during IPPV, driving pressure must be used and this requires pulmonary venous (left atrial) pressure to be measured though normally pulmonary capillary wedge pressure is used for this purpose. Estimates of PVR based only on pulmonary arterial intravascular pressure and cardiac output will be erroneous.

Increasing alveolar pressure leads to compression of intra-alveolar capillaries until, when mean alveolar pressure exceeds mean capillary pressure (referred to as zone 1), blood flow becomes minimal or ceases. With zero end-expiratory pressure the effect is minimal as lung volume returns to normal during expiration and so alveolar size and pulmonary capillary dimensions are unchanged throughout much of the respiratory cycle. Addition of PEEP leads to large increases in alveolar pressure as described above, and the resulting lung expansion will reduce PVR and introduce areas with zone 1 conditions. Animal studies, using colloidal gold particles in the circulation, have shown that with normal respiration there is perfusion in all pulmonary capillaries, including those in non-dependent areas.[16] A similar study using fluorescently labelled albumin but with airway pressure increased above pulmonary capillary pressure, showed no flow in almost two-thirds of capillaries in non-dependent regions.[17] These studies demonstrate that during artificial ventilation unperfused pulmonary capillaries do exist, but remain available for recruitment should cardiac output increase, although with low airway pressures there is probably flow in all capillaries. It is interesting to note that studies using colloidal particles during normal respiration cannot discriminate between plasma or blood flow and have led to speculation that some, *almost* collapsed, capillaries may contain only plasma ("plasma skimming") or even blood flow from the bronchial circulation.[18]

Pulmonary blood flow

In the face of an increase in PVR, pulmonary blood flow can only be maintained if the right ventricular output is sustained and pulmonary arterial pressure elevated. In practice this is rarely the case as other effects of positive pressure ventilation normally cause a reduction in cardiac output. Several mechanisms contribute to the reduction in cardiac output seen with artificial ventilation, and these have been reviewed recently.[4] The most important changes are:

- Reversal of the "thoracic pump" by which the normal negative intrathoracic pressure during spontaneous inspiration draws blood into the chest from the venae cavae, contributing significantly to venous return. With IPPV venous return *decreases* during inspiration, and when PEEP is added, venous return will be impeded throughout the respiratory cycle. The degree of impairment of venous return is in fact directly proportional to the mean intrathoracic pressure,[19] such that changes in *I:E* ratio, ventilatory pattern etc., will also affect the cardiovascular changes seen. Interestingly, these changes are mitigated to some extent during a positive pressure inspiration by diaphragmatic descent into the abdomen, which raises intra-abdominal pressure and so reduces the pressure gradient opposing flow between the abdomen and chest.[20]
- At high lung volumes, as may occur with high levels of PEEP, the heart may be directly compressed by lung expansion so preventing adequate filling of the cardiac chambers. This effect also occurs with intrinsic or auto-PEEP[15] and has been described as applying a "tourniquet to the heart".[21]
- Ventricular contractility is affected by IPPV. Elevated intrathoracic pressure directly reduces the left and right ventricular ejection pressure, which is the difference between the pressure inside and outside the ventricular wall during systole. As a result, stroke volume will be reduced for a given end-diastolic volume.

These effects of IPPV on cardiac function are very different under pathological circumstances. For example, with hypovolaemia the deleterious effects due to reduced venous return will be considerably exaggerated.

Conversely, with a failing heart, IPPV can improve cardiac output by reducing filling pressures and returning the heart to a more favourable portion of its Frank–Starling curve. Attempts have also been made to use IPPV to boost ventricular function by applying a positive intrathoracic pressure only during systole. High-frequency jet ventilation synchronised to provide inspiration only during cardiac systole has been shown to increase stroke volume in patients with impaired left ventricular performance.[22]

Transmission of airway pressure to other intrathoracic structures is affected by lung disease. The intrapleural pressure is protected from the level of intrathoracic pressure by the transmural pressure gradient of the lungs. Animal studies have shown that reduced pulmonary compliance is the main factor governing the transmission of airway pressure to other thoracic structures. With reduced compliance the effect of mean intrathoracic pressure on cardiac output is greatly reduced.[23] Patients with diseased lungs tend to have reduced pulmonary compliance which limits the rise in intrapleural pressure; therefore, their cardiovascular systems are better protected against the adverse effects of IPPV and PEEP.

Ventilation–perfusion relationships

With spontaneous respiration, the similar regional changes in ventilation ($\dot{V}$) and perfusion ($\dot{Q}$) lead to almost uniform $\dot{V}/\dot{Q}$ ratios throughout the lung, with an overall value of approximately 0.8. This is elegantly demonstrated by the multiple inert gas elimination technique (MIGET) shown in Figure 1.3.[8] Using this method, lung areas with differing pulmonary blood flow and ventilation are plotted against all possible $\dot{V}/\dot{Q}$ ratios. Areas with $\dot{V}/\dot{Q}$ ratios of zero, represent intrapulmonary shunt, and those with $\dot{V}/\dot{Q}$ ratios of infinity equate to alveolar dead space. The position of the peaks on the abscissa represents the mean $\dot{V}/\dot{Q}$ ratio for the whole lung, whilst the width of the plots indicates the degree of variability of $\dot{V}/\dot{Q}$ ratios, or $\dot{V}/\dot{Q}$ scatter. Figure 1.3a shows that under normal circumstances, almost all lung units have $\dot{V}/\dot{Q}$ ratios between 0.1 and 1.0, with minimal shunt. Anaesthesia with spontaneous ventilation (Figure 1.3b) causes a slight widening of the $\dot{V}/\dot{Q}$ distribution and a substantial increase in shunt as a result of blood flow through atelectatic lung in dependent regions.[6]

As described above, during artificial ventilation with zero end-expiratory pressure (ZEEP) there is little change in the distribution of ventilation, and at modest inflation pressures changes in perfusion are also minimal. Improved ventilation of lung areas with previously low $\dot{V}/\dot{Q}$ ratios shifts the MIGET plots slightly to the right as overall $\dot{V}/\dot{Q}$ ratio increases, but the $\dot{V}/\dot{Q}$ scatter improves (Figure 1.3c). Addition of PEEP in excess of 10–15 cmH$_2$O leads to dramatic changes in $\dot{V}/\dot{Q}$ distribution (Figure 1.3d). The shunt is improved, but reduced pulmonary blood flow as described above

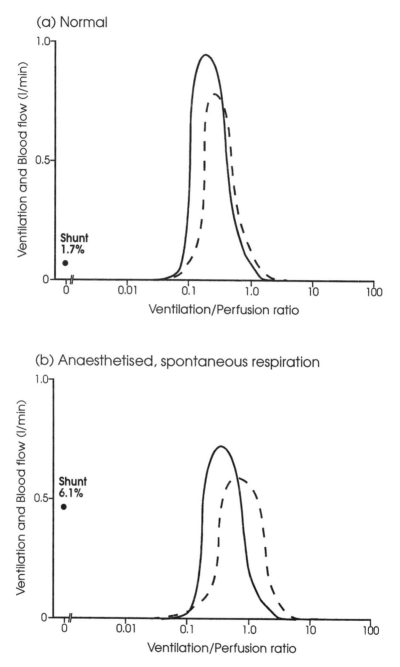

(a) Normal

(b) Anaesthetised, spontaneous respiration

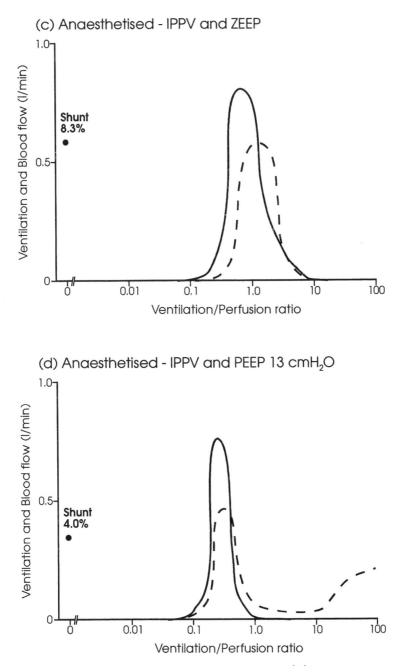

Figure 1.3   Distribution of blood flow and ventilation as a function of V/Q̇ ratios in normal subjects derived from the multiple inert gas elimination technique. See text for details. Redrawn from Bindslev LG et al., Acta Anaesthesiol Scand 1981;25:360–71, with permission.[8] IPPV, intermittent positive pressure ventilation; ZEEP, zero end-expiratory pressure; PEEP, positive end-expiratory pressure.

now causes the appearance of large areas of overventilated lung which contribute to an increase in alveolar dead space (see below).

The alterations in $\dot{V}/\dot{Q}$ distributions described in this section are unaffected by the mode of ventilation used, with MIGET giving similar results for synchronised intermittent mandatory ventilation, airway pressure release ventilation and pressure support ventilation.[24]

Dead space

Physiological dead space is defined as that part of the tidal volume which does not participate in gas exchange, and is usually expressed as a percentage of total tidal volume (V_D/V_T), with a normal value of approximately 30%. It is made up of three separate components. First, apparatus dead space is the volume of the various items of tubing and valves between the breathing system and the patient's lips. Second, the anatomical dead space, which is the volume of the conducting air passages and third, the alveolar dead space which is that part of the inspired gas which reaches the alveoli but does not take part in gas exchange. The last of these includes both ventilation to alveoli with no perfusion ($\dot{V}/\dot{Q} = \infty$) and a component due to alveoli with very high, but not infinite, $\dot{V}/\dot{Q}$ ratios.

Apparatus and anatomical dead space

Positive pressure ventilation, whether invasive or non-invasive, requires the provision of an airtight connection to the patient's airway. This inevitably involves the addition of some apparatus dead space. With orotracheal and tracheostomy tubes, much of the normal anatomical dead space is bypassed, such that any additional apparatus dead space is outweighed by the reduction in anatomical dead space. With non-invasive ventilation using face masks, apparatus dead space may be substantial. In addition, ventilator tubing used to deliver IPPV is normally corrugated, and expands longitudinally with each inspiration. For an average ventilator circuit, this expansion may amount to 2–3 ml per cmH_2O of positive pressure,[25] and this volume will constitute dead space ventilation.

Physiological dead space

In normal lungs, anaesthesia with spontaneous respiration increases V_D/V_T ratio to about 35%, and IPPV causes a further increase to around 40–50%.[8,26,27] The acute application of moderate amounts of PEEP causes a small further increase in dead space/tidal volume ratio (Table 1.1). As anatomical dead space is generally reduced, this change in physiological dead space must result from an increased alveolar component due to the increased scatter of $\dot{V}/\dot{Q}$ ratios described above. In healthy lungs, these changes do not become significant until PEEP levels exceed 10–15 cmH_2O.[8]

The alveolar component of physiological dead space may be increased substantially by ventilation of patients with acute lung injury, or when mean intrathoracic pressure is high such as with significant amounts of PEEP. Under the latter conditions, lung volume is increased to such an extent that PVR rises and cardiac output falls as described above.[28] Perfusion to overexpanded alveoli is thereby reduced and areas of lung with very high V/Q ratios develop, which constitute alveolar dead space. With IPPV in lung injury there is now good evidence that overdistension occurs in the relatively small number of functional alveoli,[29,30] and local perfusion to these lung units is likely to be impeded.

Oxygenation

Neither IPPV nor PEEP will improve arterial oxygenation appreciably in patients with healthy lungs. During anaesthesia, it has been repeatedly observed that PEEP does little to improve arterial oxygenation in the patient with sound lungs and the alveolar to arterial oxygen difference is little affected by ventilatory mode (Table 1.1). Pulmonary shunting is decreased, but the accompanying decrease in cardiac output reduces the mixed venous oxygen saturation which counteracts the effect of a reduction in the shunt, resulting in minimal increase in arterial PO_2.[8] There is however, no doubt that positive pressure ventilation improves arterial PO_2 in a wide range of pathological situations. In most cases, the improvement in PO_2 relates to the mean airway pressure achieved,[31] and, as described above, PEEP provides an easy way of elevating airway pressures. Re-expansion of collapsed lung units, improved ventilation of alveoli with low V/Q ratios, and redistribution of extravascular lung water will all contribute to the observed improvement in oxygenation.

Lung volumes and respiratory mechanics

IPPV with ZEEP will have no effect on functional residual capacity (FRC). However, with PEEP, end-expiratory alveolar pressure will equal the level of applied PEEP and this will reset the FRC in accord with the pressure/volume curve of the respiratory system (Figure 1.4). For example, PEEP of 10 cmH_2O will increase FRC by 500 ml in a patient with a compliance of 0.5 l/kPa (50 ml/cmH_2O). In many patients this may be expected to raise the tidal range above the closing capacity and so reduce pulmonary collapse. Opening of previously closed alveoli is probably the

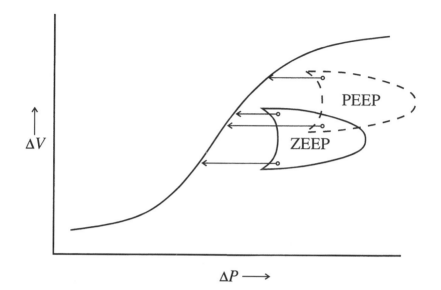

Figure 1.4 *Effect of positive end-expiratory pressure (PEEP) on the relationship between regional pressure and volume in the lung (supine position). Note that compliance is greater in the upper part of the lung with zero end-expiratory pressure (ZEEP) and in the lower part of the lung with PEEP, which thus improves ventilation in the dependent zone of the lung. Reproduced from Lumb AB. Nunn's applied respiratory physiology, 5th edn. Oxford: Butterworth-Heinemann, 1999, with permission.[14]*

greatest single advantage of IPPV and PEEP. It will also reduce airway resistance according to the inverse relationship between lung volume and airway resistance. It may also change the relative compliance of the upper and lower parts of the lung (Figure 1.4), thereby improving the ventilation of the dependent overperfused parts of the lung.

With IPPV in disease states, the effects on compliance and resistance are extremely variable. Abdominal distension and other causes of reduced chest wall compliance lead to a reduction in FRC. The ensuing pulmonary collapse is harmful enough in itself for gas exchange, but the change in FRC further reduces lung compliance by shifting tidal ventilation to the lower, flat part of the normal compliance curve shown in Figure 1.4. High inflation pressures are therefore required, leading to distension of the few remaining functional alveoli, and cyclical opening and closing of lung units will occur if tidal ventilation is occurring below the subject's closing capacity. Both these events contribute to ventilator-induced lung injury and are described below.

Addition of PEEP increases end-expiratory lung volume and may reverse the changes described in the previous paragraph. However, application of excessive PEEP in an attempt to inflate areas of collapse and improve blood-gases often causes hyperinflation in regions of, or the whole of, the lung. Once again compliance is reduced as tidal ventilation approaches total lung capacity, and lung injury may be induced.

Thus in diseased lungs, a very narrow path must be followed between reduced compliance due to lung hyperinflation with PEEP on one side and pulmonary collapse, reduced compliance and airway closure on the other.

Alveolar–capillary permeability

It has been found that PEEP increases the permeability of the lung to technetium-99m-labelled diethylenetriamine penta acetic acid (99m Tc-DTPA), a tracer molecule which does not readily cross the normal alveolar/capillary membrane.[32-34] This effect appears to be related to lung volume rather than to a pressure effect on the alveolar capillary membrane. Alveolar distension causes permeability pulmonary oedema,[30] and electron microscopic studies of animals indicate that this is a direct result of damage to capillary endothelial cell junctions, often leading to detachment of cells from the basement membrane.[35] Type I alveolar epithelial cells may also be damaged. Apart from the obvious direct increase in permeability, these changes may also trigger an inflammatory response within the lung.

The relevance of these animal findings in humans is uncertain. With extreme lung distension (45 cmH$_2$O) in animal studies, alveolar flooding occurs quickly and probably results from direct trauma to alveolar structures.[30] In larger animals and humans, the permeability changes occur more slowly (over several hours) and are more likely to result from minor structural changes to the alveolar capillary membrane leading to the alterations in surfactant and lung inflammation described below. Once again, in normal lungs the degree of alveolar distension required to produce these changes is very unlikely to occur, and many healthy patients receive several hours of IPPV during anaesthesia with seemingly negligible harm.

IPPV in pulmonary oedema

Severe pulmonary oedema from pathological causes results in degrees of hypoxia which may quickly be lethal. Tracheal intubation and positive pressure ventilation is therefore commonly required, often with spectacular results. It was originally thought that the positive alveolar pressure drove the fluid back into the circulation, but evidence that pathologically increased extravascular lung water is reduced by PEEP is contradictory, with few human studies. Animal models of pulmonary oedema indicate that by increasing the lung volume, the capacity of the interstitium to hold liquid is increased.[36] Similarly, with haemodynamic pulmonary oedema in dogs, PEEP does not alter the total amount of lung water but a greater proportion is in the extra-alveolar interstitial space,[37] and lymphatic drainage is increased,[38] and so the blood-gas interface is maintained. In addition to these theoretical benefits, the success of PEEP in patients probably depends mostly on opening up alveoli which were previously not ventilated.

Pulmonary surfactant

There has been a resurgence of interest in the function of surfactant in recent years, mostly relating to the role of the surfactant proteins (SP). Approximately 2% of surfactant by weight consists of SP, of which there are four types termed A–D. SP-B and SP-C are small proteins which are vital to the stabilisation of the surfactant monolayer following its release from the alveolar epithelial type II cell.[39] SP-A, and to a lesser extent SP-D, are involved in the control of surfactant release acting via surface receptors on type II cells which exert a negative feedback on surfactant secretion and increase uptake of surfactant precursors into the cell.

Surfactant may also play an important part in the immunology of the lung.[39] The lipid component of surfactant has anti oxidant activity, so may attenuate lung damage from a variety of causes, and also suppress some groups of lymphocytes, so theoretically protecting the lungs from auto-immune damage. Both SP-A and SP-D activate alveolar macrophages and *in vitro* studies have shown SP-A to bind influenza A virus, and increase macrophage recognition of *Mycoplasma tuberculosis*, two very common pulmonary pathogens. However, the contribution of surfactant to pulmonary defences *in vivo* remains unclear.[40]

Effects of artificial ventilation on surfactant

Animal studies have demonstrated that surfactant *release* is increased by artificial ventilation,[41,42] but there is also ample evidence that surfactant *function* is reduced.[30] Excessive surfactant loss or a defect of postsecretion stabilisation of surfactant by SP therefore seems to be the problem rather than lack of surfactant production. There are three possible explanations.

First, ventilation at low lung volumes leads to abnormal compression of the surfactant layer in alveoli which are smaller than usual. A sudden and large expansion of the alveolus may then cause disruption of the surfactant layer, converting the surface active "large aggregate" form into surface inactive "small aggregates".[43,44] This property of surfactant was demonstrated *in vitro* some years ago,[45] and has more recently been demonstrated in animals *in vivo* with both normal and injured lungs. Furthermore, the surfactant dysfunction demonstrated seems to be related to larger tidal volumes and unaffected by respiratory rate or PEEP.[43,46]

14

Second, cyclical opening and closing of small airways during ventilation causes surfactant to be drawn from the alveoli into the airway,[47] thereby removing surfactant from the alveolus quicker than it can be replaced and stabilised. Animal studies have shown that surfactant dysfunction makes alveoli more susceptible to cyclical collapse,[48] and therefore further surfactant loss, and so the establishment of a vicious cycle of pulmonary damage.

Finally, the increased alveolar–capillary permeability described above leads to the presence of several proteins in the alveolus which inactivate surfactant, particularly fibrin.[49] The resultant increase in alveolar surface tension will not only affect lung compliance but will also increase local microvascular permeability so exacerbating the tendency to pulmonary oedema and alveolar collapse.

Surfactant function is therefore inhibited most by IPPV with large tidal volumes or at low lung volume, when cyclical airway closure and alveolar compression are most likely to occur. PEEP is therefore believed to prevent many of these damaging effects.

Pulmonary inflammatory cell retention

Neutrophils, lymphocytes and erythrocytes all have mean diameters in the range 4–7 μm, which is very close to the mean diameter of a pulmonary capillary (5 μm). Erythrocytes are highly deformable, with shape changes occurring during the uptake and release of oxygen, and so can squeeze through the capillary with the cell membrane in close proximity to the endothelial cell wall. Inflammatory cells are less deformable, and so take several seconds to traverse the pulmonary capillary in contrast to the erythrocyte which does so in about 0.8 s. This slow transit time for inflammatory cells is important to facilitate margination of cells involved in pulmonary defence mechanisms. Any reduction in pulmonary capillary diameter may therefore be expected to increase pulmonary inflammatory cell retention, which has indeed been demonstrated in humans following a simple Valsalva manoeuvre[50] or with the application of 10 or 20 cmH$_2$O of PEEP.[51] In rabbits, the pattern of artificial ventilation used can also influence pulmonary neutrophil influx, with high-frequency ventilation causing less activation than conventional IPPV.[52]

If the neutrophils trapped in this way have already been activated, for example, following cardiopulmonary bypass, or systemic sepsis, then lung injury could easily ensue. Even in the absence of extrapulmonary activation, structural damage to the alveolar capillary membrane or cytokines released during margination in the pulmonary capillary may still precipitate lung inflammation.

References

1 Rushman GB, Davies NJH, Atkinson RS. *A short history of anaesthesia: the first 150 years.* Oxford: Butterworth-Heinemann, 1996.

2 Guedel AE, Waters RM. New intratracheal catheter. *Anesth Analg* 1928;**7**:238–9.

3 Cournand A, Motley HL, Werko L, Richards DW. Physiological studies of the effects of intermittent positive pressure breathing on cardiac output in man. *Am J Physiol* 1948;**152**:162–74.

4 Pinsky MR. The hemodynamic consequences of mechanical ventilation: an evolving story. *Intensive Care Med* 1997;**23**:493–503.

5 Milic-Emili J, Robatto FM, Bates JHT. Respiratory mechanics in anaesthesia. *Br J Anaesth* 1990;**65**:4–12.

6 Rothen HU, Sporre B, Engberg G, Wegenius G, Hedenstierna G. Airway closure, atelectasis and gas exchange during general anaesthesia. *Br J Anaesth* 1998;**81**:681–6.

7 Gal TJ. Is glottic function the key to improved gas exchange? *Chest* 1990;**98**:9–10.

8 Bindslev LG, Hedenstierna G, Santesson J, Gottlieb I, Carvallhas A. Ventilation–perfusion distribution during inhalational anaesthesia. *Acta Anaesthesiol Scand* 1981;**25**:360–71.

9 West JB. Regional differences in gas exchange in the lung of erect man. *J Appl Physiol* 1962;**17**:893–7.

10 Guy HJB, Prisk GK, Elliott AR, Deutschman III RA, West JB. Inhomogeneity of pulmonary ventilation during sustained microgravity as determined by single breath washouts. *J Appl Physiol* 1994;**76**:1719–29.

11 Hulands GH, Greene R, Iliff LD, Nunn JF. Influence of anaesthesia on the regional distribution of perfusion and ventilation in the lung. *Clin Sci* 1970;**38**:451–60.

12 Brudin LH, Rhodes CG, Valind SO, Jones T, Hughes JB. Interrelationship between regional blood flow, blood volume, and ventilation in supine humans. *J Appl Physiol* 1994;**76**:1205–10.

13 Brudin LH, Rhodes CG, Valind SO, Jones T, Jonson B, Hughes JB. Relationship between regional ventilation and vascular and extravascular volume in supine humans. *J Appl Physiol* 1994;**76**:1195–204.

14 Lumb AB. *Nunn's applied respiratory physiology.* 5th edn. Oxford: Butterworth-Heinemann, 2000.

15 Slutsky AS. Consensus conference on mechanical ventilation, January 28–30, 1993 at Northbrook, Illinois, USA. *Intensive Care Med* 1994;**20**:64–79.

16 König MF, Lucocq JM, Weibel ER. Demonstration of pulmonary vascular perfusion by electron and light microscopy. *J Appl Physiol* 1993;**75**:1877–83.

17 Conhaim RL, Harms BA. Perfusion of alveolar septa in isolated rat lungs in zone 1. *J Appl Physiol* 1993;**75**:704–11.

18 Johnson RL, Hsai CCW. Functional recruitment of pulmonary capillaries. *J Appl Physiol* 1994;**76**:1405–7.

19 Goertz A, Heinrich H, Winter H, Deller A. Hemodynamic effects of different ventilatory patterns. A prospective clinical trial. *Chest* 1991;**99**:1166–71.

20 Takata M, Robotham JL. Effects of inspiratory diaphragmatic descent on inferior vena caval venous return. *J Appl Physiol* 1992;**72**:597–607.

21 Conacher ID. Dynamic hyperinflation – the anaesthetist applying a tourniquet to the right heart. *Br J Anaesth* 1998;**81**:116–17.

22 Angus DC, Lidsky NM, Dotterweich LM, Pinsky MR. The influence of high-frequency jet ventilation with varying cardiac-cycle specific synchronization on cardiac output in ARDS. *Chest* 1997;**112**:1600–6.

23 Traverse JH, Korvenranta H, Adams EM, Goldthwait DA, Carlo WA. Impairment of hemodynamics with increasing mean airway pressure during high-frequency oscillatory ventilation. *Ped Res* 1988;**23**:628–31.

24 Valentine DD, Hammond MD, Downs JB, Sears NJ, Sims WR. Distribution of ventilation and perfusion with different modes of mechanical ventilation. *Am Rev Respir Dis* 1991;**143**:1262–6.

25 Shneerson JM. Techniques in mechanical ventilation: principles and practice. *Thorax* 1996;**51**:756–61.

26 Campbell EJM, Nunn JF, Peckett BW. A comparison of artificial ventilation and spontaneous respiration with particular reference to ventilation–bloodflow relationships. *Br J Anaesth* 1958;**30**:166–75.

27 Cooper EA. Physiological deadspace in passive ventilation. *Anaesthesia* 1967;**22**:199–219.

28 Biondi JW, Schulman DS, Soufer R, Matthay RA, Hines RL, Kay HR, Barash PG. The effect of incremental positive end-expiratory pressure on right ventricular hemodynamics and ejection fraction. *Anesth Analg* 1988;**67**:144–51.

29 Vieira SRR, Puybasset L, Richecoeur J, Lu Q, Cluzel P, Gusman PB, Coriat P, Rouby J-J. A lung computed tomographic assessment of positive end-expiratory pressure-induced lung overdistension. *Am J Respir Crit Care Med* 1998;**158**:1571–7.

30 Dreyfuss D, Saumon G. Ventilator-induced lung injury: lessons from experimental studies. *Am J Respir Crit Care Med* 1998;**157**:294–323.

31 Gammon RB, Strickland JH, Kennedy JI, Young KR. Mechanical ventilation: a review for the internist. *Am J Med* 1995;**99**:553–62.

32 Rizk NW, Luce JM, Hoeffel JM, Price DC, Murray JF. Site of deposition and factors affecting clearance of aerosolized solute from canine lungs. *J Appl Physiol* 1984;**56**:723–9.

33 Marks JD, Luce JM, Lazar NM, Wu JN, Lipavsky A, Murray JF. Effect of increases in lung volume on clearance of aerosolized solute from human lungs. *J Appl Physiol* 1985;**59**:1242–8.

34 Nolop KB, Maxwell DL, Royston D, Hughes JMB. Effect of raised thoracic pressure and volume on ^{99m}Tc-DTPA clearance in humans. *J Appl Physiol* 1986;**60**:1493–7.

35 Dreyfuss D, Basset G, Soler P, Saumon G. Intermittent positive-pressure hyperventilation with high inflation pressures produces pulmonary microvascular injury in rats. *Am Rev Respir Dis* 1985;**132**:880–4.

36 Gee MH, Williams DO. Effect of lung inflation on perivascular cuff fluid volume in isolated dog lung lobes. *Microvasc Res* 1979;**17**:192–6.

37 Paré PD, Warriner B, Baile EM, Hogg JC. Redistribution of pulmonary extravascular water with positive end-expiratory pressure in canine pulmonary edema. *Am Rev Respir Dis* 1983;**127**:590–3.

38 Mondéjar EF, Mata GV, Càrdenas A, Mansilla A, Cantalejo F, Rivera R. Ventilation with positive end-expiratory pressure reduces extravascular lung water and increases lymphatic flow in hydrostatic pulmonary oedema. *Crit Care Med* 1996;**24**:1562–7.

39 Hamm H, Kroegel C, Hohlfeld J. Surfactant: a review of its functions and relevance in adult respiratory disorders. *Respir Medicine* 1996;**90**:251–70.

40 Mason RJ, Greene K, Voelker DR. Surfactant protein A and surfactant protein D in health and disease. *Am J Physiol* 1998;**275**:L1–13.

41 Oyarzun MJ, Clements JA. Control of lung surfactant by ventilation, adrenergic mediators, and prostaglandins in the rabbit. *Am Rev Respir Dis* 1978;**117**:879–91.

42 Nicholas TE, Barr HA. The release of surfactant in rat lung by brief periods of hyperventilation. *Respir Physiol* 1983;**52**:69–83.

43 Veldhuizen RA, Marcou J, Yao LJ, McCaig L, Ito Y, Lewis JF. Alveolar surfactant aggregate conversion in ventilated normal and injured rabbits. *Am J Physiol* 1996;**270**:L152–8.

44 Veldhuizen RA, Yao LJ, Lewis JF. An examination of the different variables affecting surfactant aggregate conversion *in vitro*. *Exp Lung Res* 1999;**25**:127–41.

45 Brown ES, Johnson RP, Clements JA. Pulmonary surface tension. *J Appl Physiol* 1959;**14**:717–20.

46 Ito Y, Veldhuizen RA, Yao LJ, McCaig LA, Bartlett AJ, Lewis JF. Ventilation strategies affect surfactant aggregate conversion in acute lung injury. *Am J Respir Crit Care Med* 1997;**155**:493–9.

47 Faridy EE. Effect of ventilation on movement of surfactant in airways. *Respir Physiol* 1976;**27**:323–34.

48 Taskar V, John J, Evander E, Robertson B, Jonson B. Surfactant dysfunction makes lungs vulnerable to repetitive collapse and reexpansion. *Am J Respir Crit Care Med* 1997;**155**:313–20.

49 Seeger W, Grube C, Gunther A, Schmidt R. Surfactant inhibition by plasma proteins: differential sensitivity of various surfactant preparations. *Eur Respir J* 1993;**6**:971–7.

50 Markos J, Hooper RO, Kavanagh-Gray D, Wiggs BR, Hogg JC. Effect of raised alveolar pressure on leukocyte retention in the human lung. *J Appl Physiol* 1990;**69**:214–21.

51 Loick HM, Wendt M, Rötker J, Theissen JL. Ventilation with positive end-expiratory airway pressure causes leukocyte retention in human lung. *J Appl Physiol* 1993;**75**:301–6.

52 Sugiura M, McCulloch PR, Wren S, Dawson RH, Froese AB. Ventilator pattern influences neutrophil influx and activation in atelectasis-prone rabbit lung. *J Appl Physiol* 1994;**77**:1355–65.

2: Non-invasive respiratory support in the intensive care unit

MASSIMO ANTONELLI

Benefits of non-invasive ventilation

The feasibility of the application of non-invasive ventilation (NIV) in selected chronic obstructive airway disease (COPD) patients has now been demonstrated in two prospective, randomised trials.[1,2] In one of the first studies of NIV application in a small group of COPD patients admitted into the intensive care unit (ICU), the results showed a beneficial effect such that the need for endotracheal intubation was avoided in some patients.[3] In a case-control study, Brochard and colleagues demonstrated that this approach to ventilatory support could reduce both the need for endotracheal intubation and the duration of hospital stay.[4] Several other subsequent studies of COPD patients demonstrated improved gas exchange, avoidance of intubation and successful patient management.[5-11]

In the first randomised, prospective study, Bott and colleagues compared NIV with conventional treatment in a group of 60 patients with acute exacerbation of their COPD.[2] NIV was administered through a nasal mask with a significant reduction in $PaCO_2$ and dyspnoea score. In addition, there was a significant reduction in mortality from 90% to 70% ($p < 0.01$).

The efficacy of NIV in patients with acute exacerbation of COPD in the intensive care unit setting has been more recently evaluated in a European prospective randomised multicentre study, coordinated by Brochard et al.[1] Eighty-five COPD patients were evaluated. Patients with cardiogenic pulmonary oedema, pneumonia or postoperative acute respiratory failure were excluded from the study. Patients were randomly assigned to receive either conventional treatment (i.e., oxygen plus aggressive medical treatment) or conventional treatment plus NIV at an initial rate zero end-expiratory pressure (ZEEP) of 20 cmH_2O. Patients who received NIV showed a significant improvement in gas exchange within only 1 hour of treatment. The group of patients randomly assigned to NIV had a significantly lower intubation rate of 26% compared to 74% in the conventional management group ($p < 0.001$), a lower complication rate ($p < 0.01$), shorter duration of hospital stay ($p < 0.02$) and lower mortality rate (9% compared to 29%, $p < 0.02$). NIV was applied for a mean duration of four days. In those patients requiring intubation, the mortality rate was similar regardless of whether patients were initially randomised to NIV or conventional treatment (27% compared to 32%, NS).

Kramer and colleagues, in another randomised study, compared NIV delivered through nasal mask, with conventional treatment, in 26 COPD patients. Despite only a slight decrease in $PaCO_2$, the authors reported a significant reduction in the number of patients requiring intubation and a significant and stable improvement in PaO_2, heart rate and respiratory rate in those patients randomised to non-invasive ventilation.[10]

Contraindications to non-invasive ventilation

NIV can be considered as a valuable alternative to conventional mechanical ventilation in the ICU setting, provided that patients have no contraindications to mask ventilatory support. The contraindications for patient selection for NIV are shown in Table 2.1. Patients with COPD and

Table 2.1 Contraindications to non-invasive ventilation

Absolute contraindications	Relative contraindications	Caution
Coma	Angina pectoris	Edentulous patients
Impaired swallowing	Recent acute myocardial infarction (< 2 weeks)	Patients with beards
Mental incapacity	Secretions (secretions may be managed with bronchoscopy during NIV)	
Uncooperative patients (COPD patients with carbon dioxide narcosis may be an exception)		
Facial deformities or acute facial trauma		
Improperly fitted mask		
Need for endotracheal intubation to protect the airways (for example, active upper gastrointestinal bleeding)		
Haemodynamic instability		
Recent oesophageal, gastric or oral surgery		

carbon dioxide narcosis represent an exception to the absolute contra-indication of non-cooperative patients. Most of these patients will improve mental function within 15–30 min of effective NIV and only a minority will subsequently require intubation.

As a general rule, NIV should be absolutely avoided in patients with cardiovascular instability (i.e., hypotension and/or life-threatening arrhyth-mia), in those patients who require endotracheal intubation to protect air-ways, or have life-threatening refractory hypoxaemia ($PaO_2 < 60$ mmHg on FIO_2 of at least 0.6). Patients with morbid obesity (> 200% of ideal body weight) or those who have unstable angina or acute myocardial infarction may be treated with NIV, but should be closely managed by experienced personnel.

Non-invasive ventilation in patients with acute respiratory failure

Following the beneficial results obtained in patients with acute exacer-bation of COPD and the promising data of a few retrospective and non-randomised pilot studies[3,12,13] in patients with acute respiratory failure (ARF), NIV is now currently under clinical evaluation as a possible alter-native to conventional mechanical ventilation with endotracheal intuba-tion, in an attempt to reduce the intubation rate during ARF. In patients with ARF, unrelated to COPD, the aim of NIV is to decrease the amount of spontaneous work of breathing and correcting the rapid shallow breath-ing always present in acute conditions. In theory, NIV can prevent respira-tory muscle fatigue and avoid the need for endotracheal intubation.

In both my own, and our and others' experience,[6] the application of NIV by facemask seems more appropriate for patients with severe hypoxaemia and tachypnoea and who breathe through the mouth. In 1989, Meduri and colleagues reported one of the first clinical applications of NIV in patients with acute respiratory failure.[3] In this study pressure support ventilation and pressure control ventilation were used via facemask in four patients affected by cardiogenic and non-cardiogenic pulmonary oedema. Good results were achieved in three of the patients. Subsequently, in a large group of patients with ARF of different aetiologies, Pennock et al. reported a successful outcome (no requirement for intubation) in 50% of the patients treated by nasal mask NIV.[13] Promising results were obtained in the subgroup of patients affected by postoperative acute respiratory failure. The same group repeated their findings in a second study,[14] always report-ing good results. Wysocki et al. reported a 47% success rate in the treat-ment of ARF patients with NIV.[15] All of these studies, however, were not controlled and non-randomised.

In a randomised controlled study of 41 non-COPD patients with ARF, patients received with facemask NIV or conventional medical therapy.[16] NIV reduced the need for endotracheal intubation, the duration of intensive care unit stay, and mortality rate, but only in those patients with hypercapnia ($PaCO_2$ > 45 mmHg). No significant differences were seen in those patients who were hypoxaemic. On the basis of these results, the authors concluded that NIV was not beneficial when used systematically in all forms of acute respiratory failure not related to COPD. This interesting study was specifically dedicated to evaluate NIV as a tool to prevent endotracheal intubation, and not as an alternative treatment for ARF.[16]

Recently, we conducted a randomised of 64 patients with hypoxaemic acute respiratory failure who had not improved with aggressive medical therapy.[17] Patients were excluded if they had COPD, were immunosuppressed, status asthmaticus, more than two organ failures or any contraindication to NIV. Patients received either facemask non-invasive pressure support ventilation with 2–3 cmH_2O continuous positive airway pressure (CPAP) or endotracheal intubation with conventional mechanical ventilation with 5 cmH_2O positive end-expiratory pressure (PEEP). The study end points were gas exchange parameters and the frequency of complications of mechanical ventilation, including pneumonia and sepsis. The PaO_2/FIO_2 ratio improved in both groups after 1 h of ventilatory support. Ten of the 32 patients receiving non-invasive ventilation required endotracheal intubation (Table 2.2). Patients treated with conventional ventilation had more frequent and serious complications (38% compared to 66%, p < 0.002). We suggest that in patients with severe respiratory distress, NIV may lead to more favourable outcomes than conventional ventilation, in the hands of experienced staff and in the setting where this technology can be rapidly and safely administered.

Non-invasive ventilation-assisted bronchoscopy in severely hypoxaemic patients

Pneumonia with severe hypoxaemia is a common complication in immunocompromised patients, such as those affected by haematological malignancies. In these subjects the possibility of an early and correct diagnosis of the causative agent responsible for lower respiratory tract infection is clearly mandatory. Unfortunately, severe hypoxaemia in non-intubated patients represents a major contraindication to both fibreoptic brochoscopy (FOB) and bronchoalveolar lavage (BAL).[18] This may result in empirically based treatment in the absence of microbiological information. We therefore recently proposed a technique in which FOB and/or BAL can be performed in severely hypoxaemic, non-intubated patients by means of pressure support non-invasive ventilation administered through a facial mask.[19] A small group of non-intubated, critically ill patients (6 male and 2 female),

Table 2.2   Efficacy of non-invasive ventilation in critically ill patients

Parameter	SAPS score < 16		SAPS score ≥16	
	Non-invasive ventilation n = 20	Conventional ventilation n = 25	Non-invasive ventilation n = 12	Conventional ventilation n = 7
Intubation avoided (%)	85	–	33.0	–
Duration of ventilation (days)	3.2 ± 3.7*	6.9 ± 6.5	11.4 ± 8.6	8.4 ± 9.9
Duration of ICU stay (days)	7.0 ± 6.7*	16.0 ± 18.0	12.8 ± 8.1	10.0 ± 14.3
Sepsis after study entry (%)	5*	32	42	43
Ventilator-associated pneumonia (%)	0*	24	8	29
Complications (%)	25*	60	58	86
Survival to discharge	90*	64	42	14

* Significantly better than in patients receiving conventional ventilation, $p < 0.05$.
SAPS: simplified acute physiology score.

most of whom were immunocompromised, with a PaO_2/FIO_2 ratio of < 100 mmHg and with the standard criteria for nosocomial pneumonia or interstitial lung disease were studied. A bronchoscopy with bronchoalveolar lavage during NIV was performed in order to identify the causative agent of pneumonia, to start appropriate early and specific treatment and hence avoid intubation. All patients were treated with NIV for 10 min before bronchoscopy was commenced, and this was continued for at least 90 min after the procedure had finished. In all patients it was possible to identify the agent responsible for pneumonia. None of the patients subsequently needed endotracheal intubation. Six out of the 8 subjects were successfully treated and discharged from the hospital. PaO_2/FIO_2 and O_2 saturation significantly improved as expected as a result of NIV treatment. This improvement was maintained over the duration of the study. $PaCO_2$, heart rate and respiration rate did not show any deterioration during fiberoptic bronchoscopy. Bronchoscopy with NIV therefore seems to be a feasible, safe and effective technique to allow an early and accurate diagnosis of pneumonia in non-intubated, severely hypoxaemic patients. The technique appears promising enough to be applied on a large scale, and may be especially useful in immunocompromised patients. At the present time, this approach has been used in more than 50 subjects in my department.

Conclusions

Despite the relatively recent introduction of NIV in ICU patients, some consensus already exists, particularly in patients with COPD. NIV can be considered as an interesting therapeutic tool both to prevent the requirement for endotracheal intubation and to deliver an artificial ventilatory support. A non-invasive approach to ventilation should always be considered when no definitive contraindication exists. However, in patients with acute respiratory failure unrelated to COPD, results are not unequivocal, despite some promising preliminary results. Prospective randomised multicentre studies are therefore now needed in these patients.

References

1 Brochard L, Mancebo J, Wysocki M et al. Efficacy of non-invasive ventilation for treatment of acute exacerbations of chronic obstructive pulmonary disease. N Engl J Med 1995;**333**:817–22.
2 Bott J, Carroll MP, Conway JH et al. Randomised controlled trial of nasal ventilation in acute ventilatory failure due to chronic obstructive airways disease. Lancet 1993;**341**:1555–8.
3 Meduri GU, Conoscenti CC, Menashe P, Nair S. Non-invasive face mask ventilation in patients with acute respiratory failure. Chest 1989;**95**:865–70.

4 Brochard L, Isabey D, Piquet J *et al.* Reversal of acute exacerbations of chronic obstructive lung disease by inspiratory assistance with a face mask. *N Engl J Med* 1990;**323**:1523–30.

5 Vitacca M, Rubini F, Foglio K *et al.* Non-invasive modalities of positive pressure ventilation improve the outcome of acute exacerbation in COPD patients. *Intensive Care Med* 1993;**19**:456–61.

6 Meduri GU. Non-invasive positive-pressure ventilation in patients with chronic obstructive pulmonary disease and acute respiratory failure. *Curr Opin Crit Care* 1996;**2**:35–46.

7 Fernandez R, Blanch LI, Valles J, Baigorri F, Artigas A. Pressure support ventilation via face mask in acute respiratory in hypercapnic COPD patients. *Intensive Care Med* 1993;**19**:456–61.

8 Amjad H, Bismar H, McClung T. Bi-level positive airway pressure (BiPAP) during acute respiratory failure with chronic obstructive lung disease (abstract). *Chest* 1993;**104**:135S.

9 Daskalopoulou E, Tsara V, Fekete K, Koutsantas V, Christaki P. Treatment of acute respiratory failure in COPD patients with positive airway pressure via nasal mask (NPPV) (abstract). *Chest* 1993;**103**:271S.

10 Kramer N, Meyer TJ, Meharg J, Cece RD, Hill NS. Randomised, prospective trial of non-invasive positive pressure ventilation in acute respiratory failure. *Am J Respir Crit Care Med* 1995;**151**:1799–806.

11 Lofaso R, Brochard L, Touchard D *et al.* Evaluation of carbon dioxide rebreathing during pressure support ventilation with airway management system (BiPAP) devices. *Chest* 1995;**108**:772–8.

12 Meduri GU, Fox RC, Abo-Shala *et al.* Non-invasive mechanical ventilation via face mask in patients with acute respiratory failure who refused endotracheal intubation. *Crit Care Med* 1994;**22**:1584–90.

13 Pennock BE, Crawshan L, Kaplan PD. Non-invasive nasal mask ventilation for acute respiratory failure. *Chest* 1994;**105**:441–4.

14 Lapinsky SE, Mount DB, Mackey D *et al.* Management of acute respiratory failure due to edema with nasal positive pressure support. *Chest* 1994;**105**:229–31.

15 Wysocki M, Tric L, Wolff MA *et al.* Non-invasive pressure support ventilation in patients with acute respiratory failure. *Chest* 1993;**103**:907–13.

16 Wysocki M, Tric L, Wolff MA *et al.* Non-invasive pressure support ventilation in patients with acute respiratory failure. A randomised comparison with conventional therapy. *Chest* 1995;**107**:761–8.

17 Antonelli M, Conti G, Rocco M, Bufi M, De Blasi RA, Vivino G, Gasparetto A, Meduri GU. A comparison of non-invasive positive pressure ventilation and conventional mechanical ventilation in patients with acute respiratory failure. *N Engl J Med* 1998;**339**:429–35.

18 American Thoracic Society. Clinical role of bronchoalveolar lavage in adults with pulmonary disease. *Am Rev Respir Dis* 1990;**142**:481–6.

19 Antonelli M, Conti G, Riccioni L, Meduri GU. Non-invasive positive pressure ventilation via face mask during bronchoscopy with bronchoalveolar lavage in high risk hypoxaemic patients. *Chest* 1996;**110**:724–8.

3:   What's new in ventilator weaning?

LAURENT BROCHARD

Introduction

Separating the critically ill patient from the ventilator is referred to as "weaning from mechanical ventilation". Use of the terminology "weaning" suggests a gradual approach to this process of separation. Recent studies have resulted in an accumulation of data on methods of ventilator weaning, leading to a considerable improvement in knowledge and a strengthening of the ability of intensive care doctors to identify the best way this process might be conducted.

Conflicting results from multicentre trials

Two rigorously conducted recent multicentre trials by Brochard et al.[1] and by Esteban et al.[2] came to somewhat different conclusions despite a similar study design. A careful look at these studies indicates that a number of important conclusions are supported by both studies, and that reasonable explanations can account for the differences between the studies. Both studies selected patients who were proving difficult to wean, based on simple clinical criteria and the ability of the patients to tolerate a 2 hour T-piece trial. The first interesting result of these two large studies was that approximately 70% of the whole population of critically ill patients who survived a period of mechanical ventilation could be easily and successfully weaned with a single spontaneous breathing trial. When those patients who were difficult to wean were randomly assigned prospectively to different protocols and different modes of ventilation, both studies found significant differences in duration of weaning and length of stay on the intensive care unit, depending on the assigned protocol. These results demonstrated that the duration of the process was dependent not only on the patient's own process of recovery but also on the protocol used to achieve ventilator weaning (Figure 3.1). Both studies also found that synchronised intermittent mandatory ventilation (SIMV) was the worst method to separate patients from the ventilator. This may be explained on

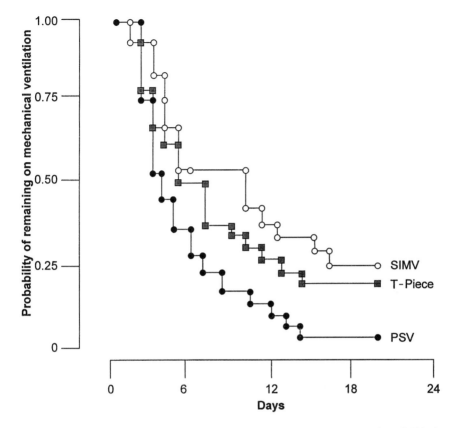

Figure 3.1   Probability of remaining on mechanical ventilation in patients with prolonged difficulties in tolerating spontaneous breathing. This probability was significantly lower for pressure support ventilation (PSV) than for T-piece or synchronised intermittent ventilation (SIMV) (cumulative probability for 21 days, $p < 0.03$). Reproduced with permission from Brochard et al.[1]

the basis of physiological studies.[3,4] The study by Brochard et al.[1] found that pressure support ventilation (PSV) was the best method to separate patients from the ventilator while Esteban et al.[2] found that a single daily T-piece trial was the most efficient method of weaning. Again, explanations for this difference may come from the specific protocols used with PSV in the two studies. Much more stringent criteria were used in the Esteban study, which resulted in a tendency to keep the patient on the ventilator longer.

A further multicentre study indirectly confirmed this hypothesis.[5] A single T-piece 2 hour trial was performed with a low level (7 cmH$_2$O) of PSV as the method of testing all mechanically ventilated patients before deciding for or against extubation. In this study, based on almost 500 patients, the same criteria were used to assess clinical tolerance in both arms of the study. The study showed that a slightly and significantly higher number of patients could be extubated from PSV than from a T-piece, although this difference was no longer significant after 48 hours.

Do we need to use protocols in the clinical setting?

Clinical judgment has often been considered to be the best method to use in deciding the right time to perform tracheal extubation. However, this has been poorly evaluated. A study by Stroetz and Hubmayr[6] showed that physicians predicted well the failure to wean, but very poorly predicted success; thus there was a strong bias towards ventilator dependency. Studies on the risks associated with self extubation reinforce this argument.[7,8] Indeed in a study by Betbesé et al. 85% of the patients who experienced self extubation did not require reintubation if this occurred when they were in the process of weaning from mechanical ventilation.[7]

Several studies demonstrated that the use of weaning protocols rather than physician-directed weaning significantly increased the rate of successful weaning, leading safely to more rapid extubation.[9,10] When the physician in charge of the patient was given the results obtained from a previous single 2 hour T-piece trial including measurement of the frequency to tidal volume ratio,[11] Ely et al. showed that this procedure significantly reduced the duration of mechanical ventilation and decreased the incidence of complications associated with extubation.

What is the risk associated with reintubation?

Hastening the process of separation from the ventilator may influence the rate of reintubation. A review of the literature shows that the reintubation rate among a population of medical and surgical critically ill patients varies from 0%[12] to 20%,[2,5] but that the usual rate is around 12–15%. Reintubation is likely to increase the risk of nosocomial pneumonia[13] but the influence on outcome remains unclear.[2,14,15] Although reintubation is associated with a poorer outcome, it seems to be more a marker of severity of illness than a contributing factor to poor outcome itself. Prediction of the need for reintubation, i.e., extubation failure, is still very difficult. Recent data obtained from studies of patients with neurological disorders in whom reintubation is often required for copious secretion, which leads to an inability to cough and protect the airways, indicate that the maximal expiratory pressure may be a useful predictor of the risk of reintubation.[16]

Conclusion

The duration and the outcome of the weaning process is heavily dependent on the way in which weaning is conducted. A systematic approach to test the ability of patients to tolerate spontaneous breathing and to reduce ventilatory support is mandatory since physicians have a natural tendency to keep patients ventilated. Both PSV and T-piece trials can be useful in this regard.

References

1 Brochard L, Rauss A, Benito S, Conto G, Mancebo J, Rekik N, Gasparetto A, Lemaire F. Comparison of three methods of gradual withdrawal from ventilatory support during weaning from mechanical ventilation. *Am J Respir Care Med* 1994;**150**:896–903.

2 Esteban A, Frutos F, Tobin MJ, Alia I, Solsona JF, Valverdu I, Fernandez R, De La Cal MA, Benito S, Tomas R, Carriedo D, Macias S, Blanco J. A comparison of four methods of weaning patients from mechanical ventilation. *N Engl J Med* 1995;**332**:345–50.

3 Imsand C, Feihl F, Perret C, Fitting JW. Regulation of inspiratory neuromuscular output during synchronized intermittent mechanical ventilation. *Anesthesiology* 1994;**80**:13–22.

4 Leung P, Jubran A, Tobin M. Comparison of assisted ventilator modes on triggering, patient effort and dyspnea. *Am J Respir Crit Care Med* 1997;**155**:1940–8.

5 Esteban A, Alia I, Gordo F, Fernandez R, Solsona JF, Rialp G, Macias S, Allegue J, Blanco J, Carriedo D, Leon M, De La Cal M, Taboada F, Gonzalez De Velasco J, Palazon E, Carrizosa F, Tomas R, Suarez J, Goldwasser RS. Extubation outcome after spontaneous breathing trials with T-tube or pressure support ventilation. *Am J Respir Crit Care Med* 1997;**156**:459–65.

6 Stroetz RW, Hubmayr RD. Tidal volume maintenance during weaning with pressure support. *Am J Respir Crit Care Med* 1995;**152**:1034–40.

7 Betbesé AJ, Perez M, Bak E, Rialp G, Mancebo J. A prospective study of unplanned endotracheal extubation in intensive care unit patients. *Crit Care Med* 1998;**26**:1180–6.

8 Chevron V, Ménard J-F, Richard J-C, Girault C, Leroy J, Bonmarchand G. Unplanned extubation: risk factors of development and predictive criteria for reintubation. *Crit Care Med* 1998;**26**:1049–53.

9 Ely EW, Barker AM, Dunagan DP, Burke HL, Smith AC, Kelly PT, Johnson MM, Browder RW, Bowton DL, Haponik EF. Effect on the duration of mechanical ventilation of identifying patients capable of breathing spontaneously. *N Engl J Med* 1996;**335**:1864–9.

10 Kollef MH, Shapiro SD, Silver P, St. John RE, Prentice D, Sauer S, Ahrens TS, Shannon W, Baker-Clinkscale D. A randomized, controlled trial of protocol-directed versus physician-directed weaning from mechanical ventilation. *Crit Care Med* 1997;**25**:567–74.

11 Yang KL, Tobin MJ. A prospective study of indexes predicting the outcome of

trials of weaning from mechanical ventilation. *N Engl J Med* 1991;**324**:1445–50.

12 Thorens JB, Kaelin RM, Jolliet P, Chevrolet JC. Influence of the quality of nursing on the duration of weaning from mechanical ventilation in patients with chronic obstructive pulmonary disease. *Crit Care Med* 1995;**23**:1807–15.

13 Torres A, Gatell JM, Aznar E, El-Ebiary M, Puig De La Bellacasa J, Gonzalez J, Ferrer M, Rodriguez-Roisin R. Re-intubation increases the risk of nosocomial pneumonia in patients needing mechanical ventilation. *Am J Respir Crit Care Med* 1998;**152**:137–41.

14 Epstein SK, Ciubotaru RL, Wong JB. Effect of failed extubation on the outcome of mechanical ventilation. *Chest* 1997;**112**:186–92.

15 Epstein SK, Ciubotaru RL. Independent effects of etiology of failure and time to reintubation on outcome for patients failing extubation. *Am J Respir Care Med* 1998;**158**:489–93.

16 Vallverdu I, Calaf N, Subirana M, Net A, Benito S, Mancebo J. Clinical characteristics, respiratory functional parameters and outcome of a 2-hour T-piece trial in patients weaning from mechanical ventilation. *Am J Respir Crit Care Med* 1998;**158**:1855–62.

4:   Positioning in acute lung injury and acute respiratory distress syndrome

ANTONIO PESENTI

Introduction

Almost all adult patients in intensive care units are managed in the supine position, largely for the convenience of medical and nursing interventions. However, although it was suggested that nursing patients with respiratory failure in the prone position may be beneficial, followed by reports of much improved oxygenation in patients with acute respiratory distress syndrome (ARDS) when they were turned from the supine to the prone position, the prone positioning is still not universally accepted.[1-4] There have been many subsequent publications in the critical care literature which address the issue of prone positioning and most of these studies show that oxygenation improves with prone positioning. However, there have also been reports which have found that occasionally oxygenation does not improve. What is most intriguing is why oxygenation should improve when patients are turned onto their abdomen. This review will describe the effects and possible explanatory mechanisms of supine versus prone positioning on oxygenation in patients with acute lung injury and ARDS.

The effect of position on oxygenation

There have been recent studies which confirm the earlier reports. In a study by Chatte and colleagues[5] the effect of prone positioning was examined in 32 patients who had severe acute respiratory failure and who were already receiving optimised mechanical ventilatory support. Patients were studied 1 hour before turning to the prone position, 1, 2, 3, and 4 hours after prone positioning, and again 1 hour after returning to the supine position. Patients were classified as responders if the PaO_2/FIO_2 ratio increased by at least 20 mmHg within 1 hour of turning to the prone position. Twenty-five patients (78%) were responders and the measures of gas exchange in 10 of these patients had returned to the levels found prior to prone positioning by the time they were returned to the supine position. However, in 13 patients the improvement in gas exchange was sustained throughout the duration of the study period ($p < 0.001$).

Similar beneficial effects were obtained by Fridrich *et al.*[6] who looked at 31 patients with ARDS following multiple trauma, using a slightly different turning regime. Mechanical ventilatory support was optimised in all patients, who were then turned to the prone position for 20 hours, followed by supine positioning for 4 hours. Patients were returned to the prone position again if clinically indicated. PaO_2/FIO_2 ratios were assessed 1 hour before turning in each case. In 6 patients the improvement was so rapid that they received only one episode of prone positioning. There was a significant increase in PaO_2/FIO_2 ratio from 126.4 (8.6) to 204.1 (19.2) mmHg [mean (SEM), $p < 0.05$] 1 hour after turning to the prone position. After a further 19 hours, gas exchange had increased and the PaO_2/FIO_2 ratio was 247.2 (17.6) mmHg ($p < 0.05$), although this had deteriorated by 3 hours after returning to the supine position (162.4 (14.5) mmHg). The pattern of improvement in gas exchange whilst in the prone position, and impairment in gas exchange when returned to supine, was maintained in subsequent cycles of turning. However, with subsequent cycles of turning there was a gradual improvement in the supine values, suggesting a gradual beneficial effect on the underlying condition.

Mechanism of the effect of position on oxygenation

Various mechanisms for the improved oxygenation have been suggested. The majority of studies have shown that improvements occur within only a few minutes of turning and are not due to either a decrease in oxygen consumption or changes in ventilator settings. The most likely explanation is modification of the mismatching of ventilation and perfusion (V_AQ) that occurs in ARDS, leading to a fall in shunt fraction (Q_S/Q_T). Ventilation is more homogeneously distributed in the prone position[7,8] and most of the change in ventilation in the prone position occurs by caudal movement of the dorsal diaphragm, which is much less mobile in the supine position.[9] Areas of underventilation in the dorsal regions are therefore recruited with little or no change in ventilation to the ventral parts of the lung. Thus the homogeneity of V_AQ is improved by decreasing the proportion of low V_AQ areas.[10-12] Gattinoni and colleagues have shown the way in which changes in body position may alter the distribution of ventilation in patients with ARDS during mechanical ventilation using the density changes generated from computed tomography (CT).[13]

The effect of position on lung density

In the supine patient with acute lung injury, CT scan shows densities at the dorsal areas of the lung, and a certain amount of preserved aeration in the ventral areas. The lung is heavy because it is oedematous – a normal lung weighs approximately 1 kg but an acutely injured lung is heavier, around 2.5 kg. This is because the injured lung is full of water, cells and proteins etc., secreted as a result of inflammation.

In the study by Gattinoni *et al.*[13] CT scans were performed in 10 patients with

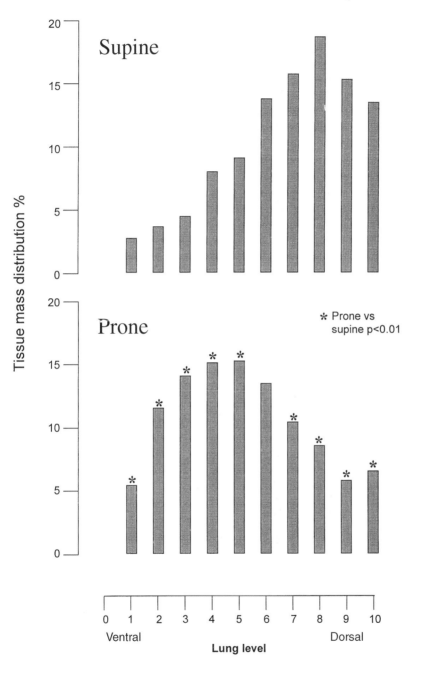

Figure 4.1 Tissue mass distribution as a function of lung level in the supine and prone positions in patients with acute respiratory distress syndrome. Redrawn from Gattinoni et al., Anesthesiology 1991;74:15–23, with permission.[13]

parenchymal acute respiratory failure in both the supine and prone positions. At equal levels of PEEP, changes in CT density in dorsal and ventral basilar lung regions induced by the change of position as well as alterations of gas exchange were measured. The CT scan image of each lung was divided into ten equal segments from dorsal to ventral. After measuring each lung fraction, the volume, the average CT number, its frequency distribution, and the expected normal value, the lung tissue mass, the excess tissue mass, and the fraction of normally inflated tissue were computed. The excess tissue mass is the amount of "tissue", which includes oedema fluid, cells and blood over and above the expected normal mass. The superimposed hydrostatic pressure on each lung region was also estimated as density × height. The authors reported that the excess lung tissue mass is similar in both the supine and prone position. However, lung CT density increased and regional inflation decreased from ventral to dorsal in both the supine and the prone positions, suggesting progressive deflation of gas-containing alveoli along the gravity gradient (Figure 4.1). This study showed that in patients with acute respiratory failure, the lung behaves like an elastic body with a diffusely increased mass.[13] Reversing gravitational forces, i.e., changing from supine to prone, induced atelectasis of previously inflated areas and inflation of previously atelectic regions, without altering the overall efficiency of oxygen exchange.

The density of the lung increases from ventral to dorsal. Effectively, the weight at each level increases on going from ventral to dorsal and the dependent lung regions are compressed by the pressure of overlying structures. The alveoli may be so compressed that these alveoli are not ventilated. Why should oxygenation improve in the prone position? We know that oxygenation takes place where ventilation occurs, not where density is. When we change the position and put the patient prone, what was dense is aerated and what was aerated is dense.

The effect of position on lung aeration

Since density increases from top to bottom of lung, then the gas/tissue ratio, which is an index of regional inflation, decays exponentially from top to bottom. There is also an exponential decay of the gas/tissue ratio, which is an index of regional inflation, from ventral to dorsal. In the supine position the gas/tissue ratio in the most ventral segment of the lung was much higher in normal control subjects than in patients with ARDS (4.7 ± 0.5 versus 1.2 ± 0.2, $p < 0.01$),[14] and this ratio decreased exponentially from ventral to dorsal, in both controls and patients with ARDS. This indicates that the volume of air decreases on going from top to bottom. In normal subjects there is more even distribution of air when lying prone than lying supine and this remains true also for the patient with ARDS. The state of aeration of the lung is more homogeneous when the lungs are prone than when the lungs are supine.

The effects of position on mechanical properties of the lung

The effects of the prone position on the mechanical properties (compliance and resistance) of the total respiratory system, the lung, and the chest wall, and the functional residual capacity (FRC) and gas exchange have also been studied.[15] In 17 normal, anaesthetised and paralysed patients undergoing elective surgery, an oesophageal balloon technique was used, together with rapid airway occlusion during constant inspiratory flow to partition the mechanics of the respiratory system into its pulmonary and chest wall components. FRC was measured by the helium dilution technique. Measurements were taken in the supine position and after 20 min in the prone position, whilst maintaining the tidal volume at 10 ml/kg, respiratory rate at 14 breaths/min and the inspired oxygen ratio at 0.4. The prone position did not significantly affect the respiratory system or the lung and chest wall compliance. Respiratory resistance increased slightly in the prone position, due mainly to the increased chest wall resistance. Both FRC and PaO_2 markedly increased from the supine to the prone position, whereas $PaCO_2$ was unchanged. The authors concluded that the prone position during general anaesthesia improved lung volume and oxygenation and did not negatively affect respiratory mechanics.[15]

In 16 patients with acute lung injury, in the prone position PaO_2 increased from a mean of 103.2 (23.8) to 129.3 (32.9) mmHg. Total respiratory system compliance, as well as end-expiratory lung volume did not change significantly. However, chest wall compliance decreased significantly from 204.0 (97.4) to 135.9 (52.5) ml/cmH$_2$O.[16] When patients are in the prone position, chest wall compliance increases and oxygenation improves, such that the bigger the change in chest wall compliance, the bigger the change in PO_2. When patients are supine, the rib cage is free to move but when the patient is prone the front of the chest cannot move as much, and most of the movement is directed towards the abdomen. The change in chest wall compliance redistributes tidal volume from the regions that are already aerated in the supine position to the base of the lung, which more reflects the physiological situation.

There are three reasonable hypotheses as to the mechanism of improvement in PO_2 and gas exchange as a result of putting the patient in the prone position. However, despite a large number of publications, we as yet have no information on how managing patients with respiratory failure in the prone position might affect outcome. A multicentre trial is now being conducted in Italy to investigate the outcome of treating patients in the prone position. The study involves 26 centres. Patients with acute respiratory failure with bilateral infiltrations and a PO_2/FIO_2 ratio of less than 200 mmHg when PEEP is at least 5 cmH$_2$O are eligible. Patients are randomised to be placed in the supine or prone position with at least 6 hours per day lying prone. If the entry criteria are still present the next day whilst the patient is supine, the patient is again placed prone. This regime continues for up to

10 days. A pilot study involving 52 patients showed that the PO_2/FIO_2 ratio improved and we await the final results of this trial.

References

1 Webster NR. Ventilation in the prone position. *Lancet* 1997;**349**:1638–9.
2 Bryan AC. Comments of devil's advocate. *Am Rev Respir Dis* 1974;**110** (suppl):143–4.
3 Piehl MA, Brown RS. Use of extreme position change in acute respiratory failure. *Crit Care Med* 1976;**4**:13–14.
4 Douglas WW, Rehder K, Beynen FM, Sessier AD, Marsh HM. Improved oxygenation in patients with acute respiratory failure: the prone position. *Am Rev Respir Dis* 1977;**113**:559–65.
5 Chatte G, Sab J-M, DuBois J-M, Sirodot M, Gaussorgues P, Robert D. Prone position in mechanically ventilated patients with severe acute respiratory failure. *Am J Respir Crit Care Med* 1997;**155**:473–8.
6 Fridrich P, Krafft P, Hochleuthner H, Mauritz H. The effects of long-term prone positioning in patients with trauma-induced adult respiratory distress syndrome. *Anesth Analg* 1996;**83**:1206–11.
7 Amis TC, Jones HA, Hughes JM. Effect of posture on inter-regional distribution of pulmonary ventilation in man. *Respir Physiol* 1984;**56**:145–67.
8 Weiner CM, Kirk W, Albert RK. Prone position reverse gravitational distribution of perfusion in dog lungs with oleic acid-induced injury. *J Appl Physiol* 1990;**68**:1386–92.
9 Krayer S, Rehder K, Vettermann J, Didier EP, Ritman EL. Position and motion of the human diaphragm during anesthesia paralysis. *Anesthesiology* 1989;**70**:891–8.
10 Pappert D, Rossaint R, Slama R, Gruning T, Falke KJ. Influence of positioning on ventilation–perfusion relationships in severe adult respiratory distress syndrome. *Chest* 1994;**106**:1511–16.
11 Beck KC, Vettermann J, Rehder K. Gas exchange in dogs in the prone and supine positions. *J Appl Physiol* 1992;**72**:2292–7.
12 Lamm WJE, Graham MM, Albert RK. Mechanism by which the prone position improves oxygenation in acute lung injury. *Am Rev Respir Dis* 1994;**150**:184–93.
13 Gattinoni L, Pelosi P, Vitale G, Pesenti A, D'Andrea L, Mascheroni D. Body position changes redistribute lung computed tomographic density in patients with acute respiratory failure. *Anesthesiology* 1991;**74**:15–23.
14 Pelosi P, D'Andrea L, Vitale G, Pesenti A, Gattinoni L. Vertical gradient of regional lung inflation in adult respiratory distress syndrome. *Am J Respir Crit Care Med* 1994;**149**:8–13.
15 Pelosi P, Croci M, Calappi E, Cerisara M, Mulazzi D, Vicardi P, Gattinoni L. The prone positioning during general anesthesia minimally affects respiratory mechanics while improving functional residual capacity and increasing oxygen tension. *Anesth Analg* 1995;**80**:955–60.
16 Pelosi P, Tubiolo D, Mascheroni D, Vicardi P, Crotti S, Valenza F, Giattinoni L. Effects of the prone position on respiratory mechanics and gas exchange during acute lung injury. *Am J Respir Crit Care Med* 1998;**157**:387–93.

5:   The early fibrotic response in acute lung injury and the role of steroids

GEOFF BELLINGAN

Introduction

Acute lung injury is a heterogeneous condition defined by the 1994 American/European Consensus Conference as a "syndrome of inflammation and increased permeability, associated with a constellation of clinical, radiological and physiologic abnormalities arising acutely after a recognised predisposing condition and not explained by left atrial or pulmonary hypertension".[1] Despite considerable effort, however, the committee could not reach a consensus on the order of events in the pathogenesis of the lung injury. It has generally been accepted that there are three phases of acute respiratory distress syndrome (ARDS) – an exudative phase, followed by a proliferative, and finally a fibrotic phase.[2,3] All investigators point out, however, that there are difficulties in such assessments because ventilator-induced injury and intercurrent nosocomial pneumonia also contribute to the gross pathological picture, which is further obscured by differences in initiating insult. One of the most consistent and striking findings in ARDS is the rapid onset of pulmonary fibrosis.[4,5] Remarkably, however, this aggressive fibrosis can resolve completely, although the mechanisms controlling both its onset and resolution are not understood. This lack of understanding of the exact pathogenesis of acute lung injury has hampered progress towards effective therapeutic interventions and despite the expenditure of many millions of dollars the development of specific therapies for ARDS has been extremely disappointing. It is becoming clear recently that despite the failure of a plethora of novel therapies, there may well be an important role for that old war horse – corticosteroids – in the treatment of ARDS. This chapter will describe our current understanding of the initiation of fibrosis in ARDS and then review the literature on the role of steroids in the treatment of ARDS.

Pathology of ARDS

One of the most prominent pathological findings in early ARDS is the eosinophilic hyaline membranes, composed of plasma proteins, mainly fibrin with some complement, that have leaked through the endothelial and epithelial lining to fill the air spaces.[4,6] This is accompanied by an inflammatory cell influx, the extent of which is related to outcome. Other early changes observed include damage to the endothelial lining, focal aggregates of neutrophils within capillaries, alveolar septal oedema, extravasated red cells and diffuse damage to epithelial surfaces with extensive type I cell necrosis.[4,5,7] In those patients who survive the initiating insult and early stages of acute lung injury, proliferative changes can then be seen in the lung. There is organisation of exudative material, proliferation and activation of type II pneumocytes and fibroblasts, and consequent elaboration of matrix proteins. Accompanying this is extensive damage and remodelling of the vasculature with occlusion of vascular intima, including small arteries, veins and lymphatics.[8,9] This proliferative phase is said to then lead onto the fibrotic phase, characterised macroscopically by coarse cobblestoned lungs with areas of scarring and areas of microcytic air spaces. By this stage there is abnormal and excessive deposition of extracellular matrix proteins, especially collagen.[5,10] Moreover, the characteristics of the fibrosis

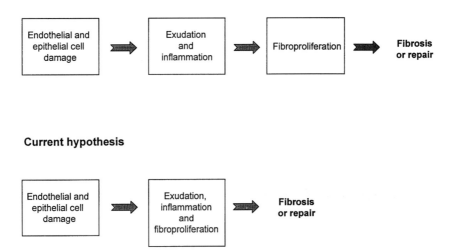

*Figure 5.1   The classical model for the pathogenesis of ARDS suggests that damage to the endothelial and epithelial surfaces leads to exudation and inflammation. Fibroproliferation then ensues, which if excessive can lead to established fibrosis. Mounting evidence suggests that fibroproliferation is an early event in ARDS, in parallel with both exudative and inflammatory events. Reproduced from Marshall et al., Thorax 1998;**53**:815–17 with permission from the BMJ Publishing group.*

in acute lung disease is similar to that seen in chronic lung fibrosis, except the time scale is enormously compressed. Total lung collagen can double in ARDS in two weeks with the fibrillar collagens – type I and III predominating.[11-13] The classical and current hypotheses of the pathogenesis of ARDS is represented in Figure 5.1.

Fibrosis in ARDS

Fibrosis in ARDS is important, as it influences outcome both directly and indirectly.[14] It reduces lung compliance, thereby increasing the work of breathing, and decreases the tidal volume, hence increasing the respiratory rate, resulting in CO_2 retention. It also reduces gas exchange because of alveolar obliteration and interstitial thickening, resulting in hypoxia. This increased compliance and the reduced gas exchange then lead to ventilator dependence. Although late deaths from ARDS may be ascribed to sepsis rather than progressive hypoxia, sepsis in these patients is usually a consequence of ventilator dependence and ventilator-associated or other nosocomial infections such as catheter-related sepsis or pressure sores.[15,16] Up to 40% of late ARDS deaths are due to progressive fibrosis and 70% are associated with nosocomial infection

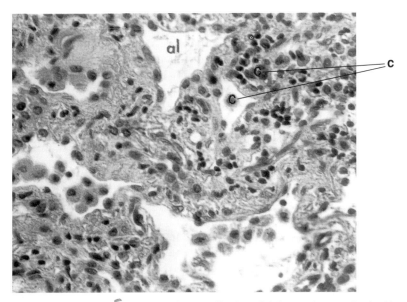

Figure 5.2   The typical histological picture of severe fibrosis and inflammation associated with ARDS demonstrating complete obliteration of alveoli (al) with compressed and collapsed capillaries (c) and an intense cellular infiltrate. Haematoxylin–eosin–saffron × 400 magnification. Reproduced with permission from Martin et al., Chest 1995;107:196–203.

and multiorgan failure. Photomicrographs showing fibrotic changes typically seen in ARDS are shown in Figures 5.2 and 5.3.

As noted by the Consensus Committee, the timing of the initiation of fibrosis is unclear, partly due to difficulties in determining the onset and progression of fibrosis. Lung biopsy is an infrequent option although it has been, along with autopsy specimens, one of the major sources of information on fibrosis in ARDS. Information on fibrosis can be gained from other sources, however. N-terminal procollagen-III peptide (N-PCP-III) is a marker for collagen turnover and there is a transpulmonary gradient for this in lungs suggesting that the lungs actively synthesise collagen III in the normal state.[17] Furthermore, N-PCP-III has been shown to be elevated both in the serum and bronchoalveolar lavage fluid of patients with ARDS, shown in Figure 5.4.[18,19] Recent studies have shown that N-PCP-III is increased within 24 hours of commencing mechanical ventilation for ARDS and that increased levels are predictive of death, such that at concentrations over 1.75 U/ml the risk of death is 4.5 times higher.[20]

There is also early evidence of increases in procollagen-I peptide levels and of myofibroblast cell numbers in alveolar walls in patients with ARDS.[21] Our studies have shown that N-PCP-III is indeed elevated within 48 hours of the initiating insult in both bronchoalveolar lavage (BAL) fluid and serum of patients with ARDS. This increase is specific to ARDS and not simply a consequence of serious illness or mechanical ventilation

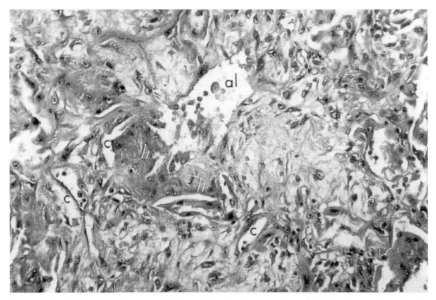

*Figure 5.3   Higher magnification of Figure 5.1. Hyaline membranes (white h) are shown in the alveolar space. Reproduced with permission from Martin et al., Chest 1995;**107**:196–203.*

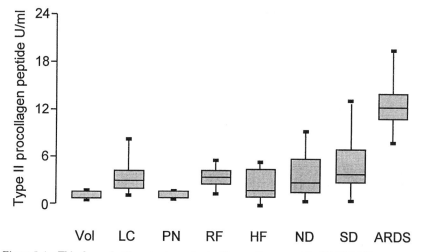

Figure 5.4   This shows significantly elevated type II pro-collagen peptide (N-PCP-III) concentrations in serum from patients with acute respiratory distress syndrome (ARDS). Volunteers (Vol), liver cirrhosis (LC), pneumonia (PN) and renal failure (RF) groups were breathing spontaneously. Heart failure (HF), neurosurgical disorders (ND), surgical disorders (SD) and ARDS groups were mechanically ventilated. Results are box and whisker plots showing median, 25th and 75th percentile and full range. Redrawn with permission from Entzian et al., Am Rev Respir Dis 1990;
***142**:1079–82.*

alone, as N-PCP-III levels were not elevated in patients ventilated for cardiogenic pulmonary oedema who had a similar APACHE score and outcome to the ARDS cohort. Moreover the BAL fluid lavaged from ARDS patients within 48 hours of diagnosis was intensely mitogenic for fibroblasts.[22] These data all suggest that the fibrosis so characteristic of ARDS may not be a late event but is switched on at a remarkably early stage of the syndrome.

Procollagen measurements reflect collagen turnover rather than deposition, and turnover is extraordinarily high, in the order of 10% of lung collagen each day. Lung collagen deposition is determined by multiple factors with fibroproliferative agents such as transforming growth factor-β, insulin-like growth factor-1, endothelin-1, platelet-derived growth factor and thrombin, all of which are capable of promoting collagen deposition. The matrix metalloproteinases (especially MMP-2 and MMP-9) and the gelatinases in contrast are responsible for collagen breakdown.[5,23,24] The roles of these mediators in ARDS are as yet quite unknown.[5] Furthermore, the massive neutrophil influx in ARDS is associated with significant elevations in pro-inflammatory cytokine levels such as tumour necrosis factor-α (TNF-α) and interleukin-1β (IL-1β) which are themselves chemotactic and mitogenic for lung fibroblasts and also stimulate collagen synthesis. Mechanical ventilation itself may be another important pro-fibrotic stimulus as abnormal shear forces developed between lung units with differing compliance can lead to exposure of basement membrane and lung injury resembling ARDS which can be compounded by oxygen toxicity.[25] It is therefore not surprising that fibrosis can be so rapid and severe in ARDS and a key question arises as to how these pro-fibrotic processes can be corrected. There is now good evidence that steroids are the first specific pharmacological therapy shown to be effective in ARDS resulting in reduced pulmonary fibrosis.

The history of steroid use in ARDS

In 1985, Ashbaugh and Maier described a good response to the use of corticosteroids in 8 out of 10 patients with biopsy-proven pulmonary fibrosis.[26] In the same year, Van Der Merwe et al. reported that in a trial of 92 patients, the early use of methylprednisolone significantly decreased the percentage of patients developing ARDS compared to controls.[27] This was contradicted by the study of Weigelt et al. which examined the role of early methylprednisolone treatment in patients with pulmonary failure, also published in 1985.[28] In this randomised double-blind trial, 81 acutely ill, mechanically ventilated patients at high risk for developing ARDS, were enrolled. Thirty-nine patients received methylprednisolone (30 mg/kg six hourly for 48 hours) and 42 received mannitol as control. Of those receiving the steroid, 64% developed ARDS with infections occurring in three-quarters. This was compared to ARDS occurring in only 33% of the controls of whom less than half developed an infection. These results clearly did not support the early use of steroids in preventing ARDS.

However, in 1986, Basran et al. published data from a small cohort of patients who had ARDS and high plasma protein accumulation in the lungs, and described a significant reduction in this protein accumulation in nearly half the patients after administration of 30 mg/kg methylprednisolone.[29] All those in whom lung protein levels fell, survived, while the mortality was over 80% in those who did not respond to steroids. The following year however, Schein et al. studied 59 patients and reported that complement pathway activation did not allow prediction of the development of ARDS and that steroid pretreatment did not influence complement levels nor prevent development of ARDS.[30]

These studies were followed by three major trials demonstrating that the early use of corticosteroids was not beneficial and may in fact be harmful, both in those patients at risk of ARDS and in those who already had early established ARDS. Luce et al. studied all patients hospitalised at San Francisco General Hospital over a three-year period who had increased temperature and decreased blood pressure but without infiltrates on chest X-ray.[31] Eighty-seven patients were randomised to receive either methylprednisolone at a dose of 30 mg/kg every 6 hours for 24 hours, or mannitol as placebo. Thirteen of the patients who received methylprednisolone developed ARDS, compared to 14 patients who received mannitol, with no differences in severity. This suggested that high-dose corticosteroid treatment was ineffective both in preventing parenchymal lung injury and in decreasing mortality in patients with sepsis syndrome. In the same year, Bone et al. investigated the early use of methylprednisolone for treatment of septic syndrome and ARDS.[32] Seventeen centres enrolled 304 patients in a prospective randomised double-blind placebo-controlled study. They identified patients with the presumptive diagnosis of sepsis, and methylprednisolone (30 mg/kg 6 hourly) or placebo was given within 2 hours of presumptive diagnosis. A trend towards increased incidence of ARDS was seen in the methylprednisolone group (32% vs. 25% $p < 0.10$) and significantly fewer patients treated with steroids had resolution of their ARDS compared with controls (31% vs. 61%, $p < 0.005$). The mortality at 14 days in the methylprednisolone group was 52% but only 22% in the placebo ($p < 0.004$). It was concluded that the early use of steroids in sepsis did not prevent the development of ARDS and indeed may have impeded the reversal of ARDS and increased the mortality.

Another prospective, randomised double-blind placebo controlled trial by Bernard and colleagues, described the use of early methylprednisolone compared with placebo in the treatment of ARDS.[33] Fifty patients received methylprednisolone (30 mg/kg 6 hourly for 24 hours) and 49 received placebo. There was no difference between groups at study entry, and after 45 days mortality was similar (60% in the methylprednisolone group and 63% in the placebo group) with no differences in reversal of ARDS or in the incidence of infectious complications. This suggested that methylprednisolone did not affect outcome in patients with established ARDS. At this stage steroids were effectively eliminated from the therapeutic armoury for patients with ARDS.

Steroids as rescue therapy in late ARDS

In 1991 Meduri et al.[34] rekindled the interest in steroids when they described a study of 9 patients with late ARDS who had fever, leucocytosis, new chest X-ray infiltrates, purulent tracheal secretions and even a low systemic vascular resistance. All patients had marked gallium uptake in the lungs but no identified source of infection. Seven of the 9 patients had open lung biopsies which showed fibroproliferation and confirmed the absence of pneumonia. Treatment with high-dose methylprednisolone was associated with a marked and rapid improvement in the lung injury score, suggesting that fibroproliferation in ARDS gives rise to clinical manifestations identical to those seen during infection, and which was potentially treatable with steroids. The authors of this study followed up their finding by

43

describing the patterns of response and predictors of outcome for use of steroids in rescue treatment of progressive ARDS, reporting on the treatment of 25 patients with a mean lung injury score of 3.[35] The average time to initiation of therapy with corticosteroids was 15 days after the commencement of mechanical ventilation. They described three patterns of response: 60% were rapid responders in whom there was a decrease in lung injury score of 1 or more, or an increase in PaO_2/FIO_2 ratio of more than 100 mmHg, in the first 7 days after steroid treatment; 24% were classed as delayed responders as they had an improvement in lung injury score or gas exchange within 14 days; 16% remained non-responders. At the time of developing ARDS no differences could be described between survivors and non-survivors and at the time of steroid treatment the only difference was that the non-survivors had a higher incidence of liver failure. Thirteen of the 25 patients had open lung biopsy which showed that preserved alveolar architecture and lack of subintimal fibroproliferation was able to distinguish between survivors and non-survivors. Responders had an 86% survival rate compared with a survival rate of only 25% in the non-responders.

Meduri *et al.* went on to examine the hypothesis that steroids were effecting patients' responses by suppressing inflammation.[36] They examined changes in TNF-α, IL-1β and IL-6 concentrations in blood and BAL fluid in response to steroids in 9 patients with ARDS, 5 of whom were rapid responders, 2 were delayed responders and 2 were non-responders. Following steroid treatment, significant reductions in TNF-α, IL-1β and IL-6 were seen in both rapid and delayed responders, although rapid responders already had significantly reduced levels of TNF-α and IL-6 at initiation of therapy.

By this stage, other investigators also began to report on the use of steroids in late ARDS. Biffl *et al.* described the survival of 5 out of 6 patients "dying" of late ARDS who were treated with methylprednisolone, and another study described a survival rate of 81% in 26 ARDS patients treated with steroids.[37]

It was suggested as a result of these uncontrolled observational studies that a sustained course of steroids may improve survival in patients with ARDS.[38] No pharmacological therapy had until this stage definitively been shown to modify the clinical course of ARDS. Meduri *et al.* therefore went on to test methylprednisolone in a randomised, double-blind, placebo-controlled four centre trial.[39] They enrolled 24 patients with severe ARDS whose lung injury score had failed to improve after 7 days. Sixteen patients were given methylprednisolone at a dose of 2 mg/kg/day for 2 weeks, after which it was slowly reduced over the next 18 days unless patients were non-responders when it was rapidly weaned. Eight patients received placebo. Those patients who did not respond after 10 days were blindly crossed to the other treatment arm. Both groups had similar lung injury score, PaO_2/FIO_2 ratio and organ dysfunction scores at study entry.

Methylprednisolone treatment however, reduced the mean lung injury score of the treatment group to 1.7 compared with 3.0 in placebo group (p < 0.001). Similarly, steroids improved the PaO_2/FIO_2 ratio (262 compared with 148, p < 0.001), decreased organ dysfunction score (0.7 compared with 1.8, p < 0.001), resulted in successful extubation (7 patients compared with none p = 0.05) and improved survival, with a hospital mortality of only 12% compared with 62% for the placebo group (p < 0.03). It was concluded that prolonged administration of methylprednisolone to patients with unresolving ARDS was associated with improvement in lung injury and organ dysfunction and reduced mortality.

The mechanism of action of steroids in ARDS

Effects on leucocyte kinetics

How do steroids work? Numerous mechanisms have been postulated. Certainly steroid treatment can prevent excessive inflammatory cell influx. However, steroids do not completely block leucocyte influx and the effect is mainly limited to studies where steroids have been used as pretreatment rather than when initiated much later after the insult. O'Leary et al. showed that pretreatment of rats with steroids reduced neutrophil influx into the lungs in a dose-dependent fashion in an endotracheal endotoxin model of ARDS.[40] The mechanism of this inhibition of cell migration is not clear, but may be more related to chemotactic signal changes than changes in adhesion molecule expression.[41,42] Certainly in vitro studies have shown that dexamethasone reduces alveolar macrophage inhibitory protein-2 (MIP-2) synthesis.

In vivo however, the effects may be different. In an intratracheal endotoxin rodent model, TNF-α and MIP-2 increased in BAL fluid with a peak at 3 hours after endotoxin challenge. Pretreatment with dexamethasone reduced TNF-α levels by 74% and reduced neutrophil influx by 58%, but had no effect on MIP-2 or on total protein influx. This suggests that those neutrophils that do extravasate potentially do so in response to MIP-2. Intratracheal endotoxin also significantly altered adhesion molecule expression on the extravasated neutrophils, with a fourfold increase in expression of the integrin CD11b but decreased expression of L-selectin in comparison to peripheral blood neutrophils. Dexamethasone had no effect on these adhesion molecule changes. Using a sheep lung lymph fistula–endotoxin model of ARDS, Lucht et al. demonstrated that endotoxin caused the release of substances into lymph that were able to stimulate neutrophils to aggregate, migrate and release superoxide.[43] This occurred within 1 hour of endotoxin and persisted for at least 4 hours. Pretreatment with methylprednisolone did not prevent the early activity but significantly reduced the activity 3–4 hours after endotoxin. Furthermore steroids can also alter leucocyte survival as they rapidly induce eosinophil and lymphocyte apoptosis but increase neutrophil survival.[44] Altering the balance of leucocyte kinetics may alter the local levels of profibrotic factors and thus effect fibrosis, or may directly improve lung compliance and outcome through a reduction in cell numbers and inflammation.

Effects on pro-inflammatory mediator cascades

Steroids can also alter inflammatory cell function, reducing levels of many inflammatory mediators and thus limiting inflammation and/or fibrosis through a dampening of these mediator cascades. Yi et al. also used an intratracheal endotoxin model in which there was increased plasma protein influx into the air spaces, along with increased neutrophil and lymphocytes emigration and increased pro-inflammatory cytokine levels.[45] These workers showed that dexamethasone reduced the protein leak, the leucocyte influx and the levels of TNF-α, IL-1β, IL-6, MIP-1α, MIP-2 and monocyte chemotactic protein (MCP-1). They concluded that corticosteroids inhibit both the vascular and cellular aspects of acute inflammation by downregulating a broad spectrum of both inflammatory cytokines and chemokines. Not only do steroids reduce cytokine and chemokine release but they can reduce arachidonic acid metabolites. Olson et al. gave intravenous E. coli to pigs, one group of which were pretreated with dexamethasone, and examined the role of leukotriene B[4] (LTB[4]) in the development of acute lung injury.[46] LTB[4] was increased 2 hours after E. coli infusion and dexamethasone significantly decreased both the haemodynamic abnormalities and BAL fluid LTB[4] levels. Similarly, Harvey et al. showed that methylprednisolone could reduce thromboxane B2 although not to the same degree as ibuprofen.[47]

Effects on pulmonary mechanics

Steroids have other beneficial effects on the lungs, including effects on airways and compliance. For example, steroids were able to inhibit free radical-induced bronchoconstriction and vasodilatation in isolated rat lungs whilst nebulised beclomethasone dipropionate prevented a decline in PaO$_2$, oxygen delivery and lung compliance over 6 hours in a septic pig model.[48,49] Grunze et al. looked at the effect of steroids on pressure–volume curves in rats challenged with bleomycin. The most significant decreases in compliance were at day 3, the time of peak inflammation.[50] Dexamethasone significantly inhibited these decreases in compliance but interestingly, methylprednisolone did not, although both steroids significantly inhibited inflammation histologically.

46

Critical importance of timing of steroids

The timing of corticosteroids are important however, as we have seen, and this is emphasised in the study by Chiara *et al.* who gave intraperitoneal zymosan to rabbits resulting in hypoxia, interstitial alveolar oedema and superoxide formation in the lungs.[51] Methylprednisolone pretreatment prevented this, but if the steroid was given 24 hours after zymosan, it had no effect. Borg *et al.* looked at both prophylactic and delayed treatment with high doses of methylprednisolone in a porcine endotoxin model of early ARDS.[52] Pretreatment with steroids prevented impairment of gas exchange and pulmonary oedema. The fall in circulating neutrophil numbers induced by endotoxin was also prevented, although there was still a substantial accumulation of neutrophils within the lungs. Pretreatment with steroids resulted in improved survival in this model. If methylprednisolone was given 2 hours after, rather than before, the injury it could prevent further deterioration in gas exchange and reduce pulmonary oedema but had no effect on circulating or extravasated neutrophil numbers.

Direct effect of steroids on matrix protein metabolism

It is known that steroids have direct effects on matrix protein metabolism as they selectively decrease cellular collagen synthesis, compared with non-collagen protein synthesis, by reducing translatable levels of mRNA for procollagens. Oikarinen *et al.* investigated the effects of topical steroids in healthy skin, examining collagen pro-peptide levels, collagen mRNA level, and matrix metalloproteinase (MMP)-1 and MMP-2 mRNA levels in human skin.[53] Treatment of healthy skin for 3 days with topical betamethasone caused a 70–80% decrease in type I and III collagen pro-peptides, indicating that the decrease in collagen synthesis after topical glucocorticoid treatment is apparently due to a decrease in corresponding mRNA. Collagen crosslinking and degrading enzymes were not decreased in the same skin samples. This suggests that *in vivo*, glucocorticoids variably modulate the genes involved in collagen synthesis and degradation.

Conclusion

Which or how many of these many potential mechanisms are involved in the therapeutic effects of steroids in late ARDS is not known. Neither do we understand whether the beneficial effects result from the influence of steroids on the inflammatory response or if it is their direct effect on collagen metabolism. These all deserve further investigation so that the optimal timing, doses and route of delivery can be established and the potential for more focused therapy can be delineated. We should also consider whether the fibrosis in ARDS is a potential model for other pulmonary fibrotic conditions and if this gives us further insights into treatment of fibrotic conditions in general.

References

1 Bernard GR, Artigas A, Brigham KL, Carlet J, Falke K, Hudson L, Lamy M, Legall JR, Morris A, Spragg R and the consensus committee. The American–European consensus conference on ARDS. Definitions, mechanisms, relevant outcomes and clinical trial co-ordination. *Am J Respir Crit Care* 1994;**149**:818–24.

2 Katzenstein AL, Bloor CM, Leibow AA. Diffuse alveolar damage – the role of oxygen, shock, and related factors. A review. *Am J Pathol* 1976;**85**:209–28.

3 Pratt PC, Vollmer RT, Shelburne JD, Crapo JD. Pulmonary morphology in a multihospital collaborative extracorporeal membrane oxygenation project. I. Light microscopy. *Am J Pathol* 1976;**95**:191–214.

4 Fukuda Y, Ishizaki M, Masuda Y, Kimura G, Kawanami O, Masugi Y. The role of intraalveolar fibrosis in the process of pulmonary structural remodeling in patients with diffuse alveolar damage. *Am J Pathol* 1987;**126**:171–82.

5 Marshall R, Bellingan G, Laurent G. The acute respiratory distress syndrome: fibrosis in the fast lane. *Thorax* 1998;**53**:815–17.

6 Rinaldo JE, Rogers RM. Adult respiratory-distress syndrome: changing concepts of lung injury and repair. *N Engl J Med* 1982;**306**:900–9.

7 Luce JM. Acute lung injury and the acute respiratory distress syndrome. *Crit Care Med* 1998;**26**:369–76.

8 Snow RL, Davies P, Pontoppidan H, Zapol WM, Reid L. Pulmonary vascular remodeling in adult respiratory distress syndrome. *Am Rev Respir Dis* 1982;**26**:887–92.

9 Zapol WM, Snider MT. Pulmonary hypertension in severe acute respiratory failure. *N Engl J Med* 1977;**296**:476–80.

10 Zapol WM, Trelstad RL, Coffey JW, Tsai I, Salvador RA. Pulmonary fibrosis in severe acute respiratory failure. *Am Rev Respir Dis* 1979;**119**:547–54.

11 Farjanel J, Hartmann DJ, Guidet B, Luquel L, Offenstadt G. Four markers of collagen metabolism as possible indicators of disease in the adult respiratory distress syndrome. *Am Rev Respir Dis* 1993;**147**:1091–9.

12 Raghu G, Striker LJ, Hudson LD, Striker GE. Extracellular matrix in normal and fibrotic human lungs. *Am Rev Respir Dis* 1985;**131**:281–9.

13 Kirk JM, Heard BE, Kerr I, Turner-Warwick M, Laurent GJ. Quantitation of types I and III collagen in biopsy lung samples from patients with cryptogenic fibrosing alveolitis. *Coll Relat Res* 1984; **4**:169–82.

14 Martin C, Papazian L, Payan MJ, Saux P, Gouin F. Pulmonary fibrosis correlates with outcome in adult respiratory distress syndrome. A study in mechanically ventilated patients. *Chest* 1995;**107**:196–200.

15 Montgomery AB, Stager MA, Carrico CJ, Hudson LD. Causes of mortality in patients with the adult respiratory distress syndrome. *Am Rev Respir Dis* 1985;**132**:485–9.

16 Bell RC, Coalson JJ, Smith JD, Johanson WG Jr. Multiple organ system failure and infection in adult respiratory distress syndrome. *Ann Intern Med* 1983;**99**:293–8.

17 Harrison NK, Laurent GJ, Evans TW. Transpulmonary gradient of type III procollagen peptides: acute effects of cardio-pulmonary bypass. *Intensive Care Med* 1992;**18**:290–2.

18 Entzian P, Huckstadt A, Kreipe H, Barth J. Determination of serum concentrations of type III procollagen peptide in mechanically ventilated patients. Pronounced augmented concentrations in the adult respiratory distress syndrome. *Am Rev Respir Dis* 1990;**142**:1079–82.

19 Clark JG, Milberg JA, Steinberg KP, Hudson LD. Type III procollagen peptide in the adult respiratory distress syndrome. Association of increased peptide levels in bronchoalveolar lavage fluid with increased risk for death. *Ann Intern Med* 1995;**122**:17–23.

20 Chesnutt AN, Matthay MA, Tibayan FA, Clark JG. Early detection of type III procollagen peptide in acute lung injury. Pathogenetic and prognostic significance. *Am J Respir Crit Care Med* 1997; **156**:840–5.

21 Liebler JM, Qu Z, Buckner B, Powers MR, Rosenbaum JT. Fibroproliferation and mast cells in the acute respiratory distress syndrome. *Thorax* 1998;**53**:823–9.

22 Marshall, RP, Bellingan GJ, Puddicome A, Goldsack N, Chambers R, McAnulty R, Laurent GJ. Early fibroproliferation in the acute respiratory distress syndrome (abstract). *Am J Respir Crit Care Med* 1999; **159**:A378.

23 Torii K, Iida K, Miyazaki Y, Saga S, Kondoh Y, Taniguchi H, Taki F, Takagi K, Matsuyama M, Suzuki R. Higher concentrations of matrix metalloproteinases in bronchoalveolar lavage fluid of patients with adult respiratory distress syndrome. *Am J Respir Crit Care Med* 1997;**155**:43–6.

24 Delclaux C, D'Ortho MP, Delacourt C, Lebargy F, Brun-Buisson C, Brochard L, Lemaire F, Lafuma C, Harf A. Gelatinases in epithelial lining fluid of patients with adult respiratory distress syndrome. *Am J Physiol* 1997;**272**:L442–51.

25 Dreyfuss D, Soler P, Basset G, Saumon G. High inflation pressure pulmonary edema. Respective effects of high airway pressure, high tidal volume, and positive end-expiratory pressure. *Am Rev Respir Dis* 1988;**137**:1159–64.

26 Ashbaugh DG, Maier RV. Idiopathic pulmonary fibrosis in adult respiratory distress syndrome. Diagnosis and treatment. *Arch Surg* 1985;**120**:530–5.

27 Van Der Merwe CJ, Louw AF, Welthagen D, Schoeman HS. Adult respiratory distress syndrome in cases of severe trauma – the prophylactic value of methylprednisolone sodium succinate. *S Afr Med J* 1985;**67**:279–84.

28 Weigelt JA, Norcross JF, Borman KR, Snyder WH III. Early steroid therapy for respiratory failure. *Arch Surg* 1985;**120**:536–40.

29 Basran GS, Byrne AJ, Hardy JG, Richardson MA. The effect of methylprednisolone on the pulmonary accumulation of transferrin in the adult respiratory distress syndrome. *Eur J Respir Dis* 1986;**68**:336–41.

30 Schein RM, Bergman R, Marcial EH, Schultz D, Duncan RC, Arnold PI, Sprung CL. Complement activation and corticosteroid therapy in the development of the adult respiratory distress syndrome. *Chest* 1987;**91**:850–4.

31 Luce JM, Montgomery AB, Marks JD, Turner J, Metz CA, Murray JF. Ineffectiveness of high-dose methylprednisolone in preventing parenchymal lung injury and improving mortality in patients with septic shock. *Am Rev Respir Dis* 1988;**138**:62–8.

32 Bone RC, Fisher CJ Jr, Clemmer TP, Slotman GJ, Metz CA. Early methylprednisolone treatment for septic syndrome and the adult respiratory distress syndrome. *Chest* 1987;**92**:1032–6.

33 Bernard GR, Luce JM, Sprung CL, Rinaldo JE, Tate RM, Sibbald WJ, Kariman K, Higgins S, Bradley R, Metz CA *et al*. High-dose corticosteroids in patients with the adult respiratory distress syndrome. *N Engl J Med* 1987;**317**:1565–70.

34 Meduri GU, Belenchia JM, Estes RJ, Wunderink RG, El Torky M, Leeper KV Jr. Fibroproliferative phase of ARDS. Clinical findings and effects of corticosteroids *Chest* 1991;**100**:943–52.

35 Meduri GU, Chinn AJ, Leeper KV, Wunderink RG, Tolley E, Winer-Muram HT, Khare V, Eltorky M. Corticosteroid rescue treatment of progressive fibroproliferation in late ARDS. Patterns of response and predictors of outcome. *Chest* 1994;**105**:1516–27.

36 Meduri GU, Headley S, Tolley E, Shelby M, Stentz F, Postlethwaite A. Plasma and BAL cytokine response to corticosteroid rescue treatment in late ARDS. *Chest* 1995;**108**:1315–25.

37 Biffl WL, Moore FA, Moore EE, Haenel JB, McIntyre RC Jr, Burch JM. Are corticosteroids salvage therapy for refractory acute respiratory distress syndrome? *Am J Surg* 1995;**170**:591–5.

38 Hooper RG, Kearl RA. Established adult respiratory distress syndrome successfully treated with corticosteroids. *S Afr Med J* 1996;**89**:359–64.

39 Meduri GU, Headley AS, Golden E, Carson SJ, Umberger RA, Kelso T, Tolley EA. Effect of prolonged methylprednisolone therapy in unresolving acute respiratory distress syndrome: a randomized controlled trial. *JAMA* 1998;**280**:159–65.

40 O'Leary EC, Evans GF, Zuckerman SH. In vivo dexamethasone effects on neutrophil effector functions in a rat model of acute lung injury. *Inflammation* 1997;**21**:597–608.

41 O'Leary EC, Zuckerman SH. Glucocorticoid-mediated inhibition of neutrophil emigration in an endotoxin-induced rat pulmonary inflammation model occurs without an effect on airways MIP–2 levels. *Am J Respir Cell Mol Biol* 1997;**16**:267–74.

42 O'Leary EC, Marder P, Zuckerman SH. Glucocorticoid effects in an endotoxin-induced rat pulmonary inflammation model: differential effects on neutrophil influx, integrin expression, and inflammatory mediators. *Am J Respir Cell Mol Biol* 1996;**15**:97–106.

43 Lucht WD, Bernard GR, Butka B, Brigham KL. Corticosteroids inhibit endotoxin-induced lung lymph neutrophil stimulating activity in sheep. *Am J Med Sci* 1988; **296**:98–102.

44 Meagher LC, Cousin JM, Seckl JR, Haslett C. Opposing effects of glucocorticoids on the rate of apoptosis in neutrophilic and eosinophilic granulocytes. *J Immunol* 1996;**156**:4422–8.

45 Yi ES, Remick DG, Lim Y, Tang W, Nadzienko CE, Bedoya A, Yin S, Ulich TR. The intratracheal administration of endotoxin: X. Dexamethasone downregulates neutrophil emigration and cytokine expression *in vivo*. *Inflammation* 1996;**20**:165–75.

46 Olson NC, Dobrowsky RT, Fleisher LN. Dexamethasone blocks increased leukotriene B[4] production during endotoxin-induced lung injury. *J Appl Physiol* 1988;**64**:2100–7.

47 Harvey CF, Sugerman HJ, Tatum JL, Sielaff TD, Lee EC, Blocher CR. Ibuprofen and methylprednisolone in a pig *Pseudomonas* ARDS model. *Circ Shock* 1987;**21**:175–83.

48 Kjaeve J, Ingebrigtsen T, Naess L, Bjertnaes L, Vaage J. Methylprednisolone attenuates airway and vascular responses induced by reactive oxygen species in isolated, plasma-perfused rat lungs. *Free Rad Res* 1996;**25**:407–14.

49 Walther S, Jansson I, Berg S, Olsson Rex L, Lennquist S. Corticosteroid by aerosol in septic pigs—effects on pulmonary function and oxygen transport. *Intensive Care Med* 1993;**19**:155–60.

50 Grunze MF, Parkinson D, Sulavik SB, Thrall RS. Effect of corticosteroids on lung volume-pressure curves in bleomycin-induced lung injury in the rat. *Exp Lung Res* 1988;**14**:183–95.

51 Chiara O, Giomarelli PP, Borrelli E, Casini A, Segala M, Grossi A. Inhibition by methylprednisolone of leukocyte-induced pulmonary damage. *Crit Care Med* 1991;**19**:260–5.

52 Borg T, Gerdin B, Modig J. Prophylactic and delayed treatment with high-dose methylprednisolone in a porcine model of early ARDS induced by endotoxaemia. *Acta Anaesthesiol Scand* 1985;**29**:831–45.

53 Oikarinen A, Haapasaari KM, Sutinen M, Tasanen K. The molecular basis of glucocorticoid-induced skin atrophy: topical glucocorticoid apparently decreases both collagen synthesis and the corresponding collagen mRNA level in human skin *in vivo*. *Br J Dermatol* 1998;**139**:1106–10.

6: Capillary stress failure and pulmonary damage*

JOHN B WEST

Introduction

The pulmonary blood-gas barrier must be extremely thin for gas exchange to take place, but must also be very strong to cope with the stresses posed by high capillary pressures. Stress failure of the capillaries results in several pathological conditions and this review will address some of the conditions relevant to intensive care.

The first reference to the blood-gas barrier was made in 1661, when the whole mass of the lung was described under light microscopy, as an aggregate of very thin fine membranes. Although the light microscope improved, with better resolution images, in fact relatively little further progress was made with regard to the blood-gas barrier, as it was at the limit of resolution of the light microscope. In 1929, a French physiologist described the respiratory surface as being similar to the flesh of an open wound. In other words, it was thought that the only thing that separated the blood from the air in the lungs was the capillary endothelium. The structure of the blood-gas barrier remained just beyond the resolution of the light microscope such that the structure could not be clearly observed. However, with the introduction of the electron microscope, the blood-gas barrier was able to be visualised with considerable clarity. The first electron micrograph of the blood-gas barrier in the lung was produced by Frank Low. It was then possible to see the capillary lumen, the alveolar space, the nucleus of the type I alveolar epithelial cell, the endothelium and the extracellular matrix which separates the two cellular layers. It was quite clear then that there were three layers in the blood-gas barrier. Of course, modern electron microscopes reveal the blood-gas barrier with exquisite detail.

Very often the pulmonary capillary in the human lung is polarised in the sense that one side of the capillary is thinner than the other. The thin side has three layers, the alveolar epithelium, the capillary endothelium and the extracellular matrix, which is made up of a fused basement membrane of the two cellular layers. On the thick side there are other structures in addi-

* This chapter is based on the 1998 Gillian Hanson Lecture.

tion, including type I collagen and other cell types. It is thought that the thinner side is mainly used for gas exchange since exchange of oxygen and carbon dioxide in the lung is by passive diffusion and it is therefore essential to have an extremely thin blood-gas barrier. The thicker side is probably the site of fluid exchange. In fact, in the early stages of pulmonary oedema it has been shown that all escape of fluid occurs on the thicker side of the blood-gas barrier with apparently very little escaping on the thinner side.

The blood-gas barrier

The thin side of the blood-gas barrier is excruciatingly thin. In the human lung it is of the order of 0.2–0.4 μm.[1] In comparison, red blood cells have a diameter of about 7 μm, which puts the depth of the blood-gas barrier into context. In a series of studies using anaesthetised rabbits, the pulmonary artery and the left atrium were cannulated and the lung was perfused at varying capillary perfusion pressures.[2,3] The capillary transmural pressure, which is the pressure difference between the inside and the outside of the capillary, was measured. The capillaries were perfusion-fixed with glutaraldehyde, enabling visualisation of the ultrastructure using electron microscopy. When the capillary perfusion pressure reached 24 mmHg, some disruption of the capillary endothelial layer or alveolar epithelial layer was observed. Usually the basement membrane remained intact. At

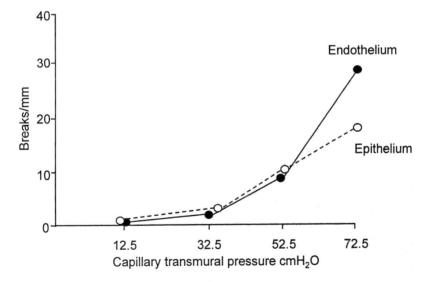

Figure 6.1   The effect of raising pulmonary capillary pressure on the number of breaks in the endothelium and epithelium. Reproduced with permission from Tsukimoto et al., 1991.[3]

pressures over 39 mmHg, consistent ultrastructural changes were seen, resulting in high permeability oedema and alveolar haemorrhage. The relationship between capillary transmural pressure and the frequency of endothelium and epithelial disruption is shown in Figure 6.1.

The exposed basement membrane which results is highly reactive due to its electrical charge such that platelets, red blood cells and leucocytes are frequently seen apparently adherent to the exposed membrane. Scanning electron microscopy (Figure 6.2) reveals the view which would be obtained from inside the alveolus looking at the wall of the alveolus. The reason

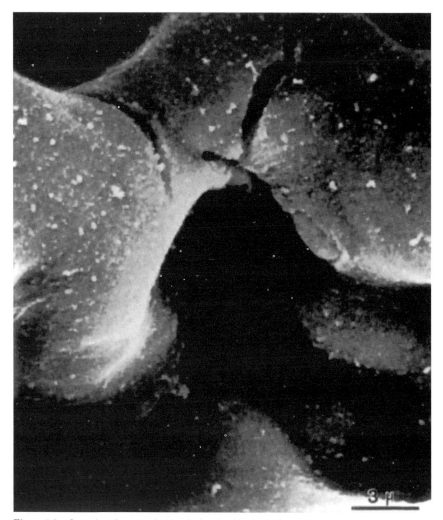

Figure 6.2 Scanning electron micrograph showing breaks in the alveolar epithelium as a result of stress failure of pulmonary capillaries. Reproduced with permission from Costello et al., 1992.[25]

these disruptions of both the endothelial and epithelial layers occur when the capillary pressure or the capillary transmural pressure is raised is relatively simple. By raising the pressure, the hoop or circumferential stress in the capillary is increased. The capillary is a thin walled tube like a garden hose – if you stand on the end of a garden hose when it is switched on the garden hose will expand, or even rupture, due to the increase in the hoop or circumferential stress in the thin-walled chamber. The diameter of the capillary is relatively low, and according to the Laplace relationship,[2] this will reduce the capillary wall stress. However, although the diameter of the capillary is approximately 5 μm, the wall thickness is only in the region of 0.2 μm, necessary for gas exchange, and consequently stress failure may result.

Capillary wall stress

There are two ways of increasing the stress in the capillary wall. The pressure inside the capillary can be raised, increasing the circumferential stress. Increased lung volume will have a similar effect, since under these conditions the tension in the alveolar wall is increased and some of this tension is transmitted to the walls of capillaries. This happens at high lung volumes where there is very good evidence that the tension in alveolar walls is greatly increased. The alveolar wall is basically a string of capillaries, which make up the alveolar wall. Therefore it is not surprising that if the tension in the alveolar wall is increased at high states of lung inflation, for example, high levels of positive end-expiratory pressure (PEEP), then the stress in the capillary wall is also raised.

Structure of the alveolar basement membrane

The blood-gas barrier is vulnerable to stress failure when capillary pressure rises. The thin side of the barrier consists of the capillary endothelial layer, the alveolar epithelial layer and the extracellular matrix, which is made up of the fused basement membranes of the two cellular layers. There is very good evidence that the strength of the capillary wall comes from the extracellular matrix, specifically the type IV collagen in the basement membranes. The principal components of the alveolar basement membrane comprise four main molecules: type IV collagen, which is enormously strong in the same way as type I collagen, which is itself responsible for probably the strongest soft tissues in the body, including the Achilles tendon; a molecule called laminin which links basement membrane to overlying cells; heparan sulphate proteoglycans which form a charge shield and regulate, to some extent, permeability of the blood-gas barrier, although this has never been proven. In addition, there is a molecule called entactin, or nidogen, which binds laminin to type IV collagen. Type IV collagen is an interesting molecule about 400 nm long, comprising a triple helix. Two molecules join at the C-terminal end and four join at the N-terminal ends to give a lattice-type appearance resembling chicken wire.[4] This structure apparently combines great strength with porosity, and studies have shown that the tensile strength of basement membranes is similar to that of type IV collagen, suggesting that it is this molecule which is responsible for the strength of the capillary wall.

There is evidence that the type IV collagen is not uniformly distributed throughout the extracellular matrix. Electron microscopy reveals that the extracellular matrix has a central lamina densa, and on the epithelial side there is the lamina rara externa and on the inside the lamina rara interna. Immunostaining has shown that most of the type IV collagen is associated with the lamina densa, right in the centre of the thin side of the blood-gas barrier (Figure 6.3). The thickness of the lamina densa is approximately 0.05 μm, or 50 nm. This very thin band is the lifeline which is protecting against rupture of the blood-gas barrier. Obviously leaking fluid or blood into the alveolar spaces would be catastrophic for gas exchange which emphasises the extreme importance of this structure.

Increased capillary pressure

There are a number of pathological conditions in which stress failure of pulmonary capillaries is involved (Table 6.1).

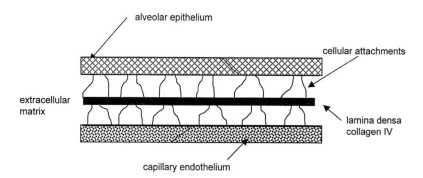

Figure 6.3   Schematic diagram showing the structure of the thin part of the blood gas barrier/lamina densa in the centre of the extracellular matrix contains most of the type IV collagen which is thought to give the barrier its strength. Reproduced from West JB, Mathieu-Costello O. Strength of the pulmonary blood gas barrier. Resp Physiol 1992;88:141–8 with permission from Elsevier Science.[26]

Table 6.1 Clinical conditions in which stress failure of pulmonary capillaries is implicated. Reproduced with permission from West JB, Mathieu-Costello O. Vulnerability of pulmonary capillaries in heart disease. *Circulation* 1995; **92**: 622–31.[27]

Increased capillary pressure and high-permeability oedema	Neurogenic pulmonary oedema High-altitude pulmonary oedema Some cases of ARDS
Increased capillary pressure causing alveolar haemorrhage	Exercise-induced pulmonary haemorrhage in racehorses Bleeding in elite human athletes Catastrophic increase in pulmonary venous pressure
Increased capillary pressure causing oedema and haemorrhage	Chronic venous hypertension, e.g. mitral stenosis Haemorrhagic pulmonary oedema in elite human athletes
Volume trauma	High PEEP levels in ventilated patients
Structural failure of the capillary wall	Goodpasture's syndrome

Pulmonary oedema can be classified as increased capillary pressure (hydrostatic or cardiogenic oedema) or increased permeability of the capillary walls (high-permeability oedema). The distinction between these two classifications has usually been on the basis of the protein concentration of the oedema fluid.[5] The differences occur because the blood-gas barrier tends to retain its low-permeability functions in hydrostatic oedema, but damage to the capillary wall increases its permeability leading to increased protein losses. In practice, distinguishing these classifications on the basis of protein loss is not conclusive, and animal studies have shown that there is a spectrum of types of pulmonary oedema as capillary pressure rises.[2]

If the capillary wall is damaged, a high-permeability type of oedema is expected because protein and cells will leak into the alveolar spaces. Neurogenic pulmonary oedema and high-altitude pulmonary oedema are conditions where the increase in capillary pressure causes a high-permeability type of oedema. There is another very interesting set of conditions where increased capillary pressure causes haemorrhage in the lungs. Racehorses very quickly develop exercise-induced pulmonary haemorrhage and even extreme exercise in humans will result in a similar phenomenon. Increased pressure can also cause a combination of oedema and haemorrhage, such as is seen in mitral stenosis when haemoptysis occurs and the lungs are haemosiderin loaded, and pulmonary oedema results. Overinflation of the lungs is an important cause of morbidity in the intensive care unit, and this condition will be also be discussed.

Neurogenic pulmonary oedema

Neurogenic pulmonary oedema has been studied extensively due to its importance in cranial injury from trauma. Patients may be admitted onto intensive care units with severe head injury and quickly go on to develop pulmonary oedema and all its consequences. It has been shown both experimentally and also in patients, that neurogenic pulmonary oedema is associated with extremely high pulmonary arterial and wedge pressures.[6,7] In fact it has been shown that these high pressures are associated with greatly increased levels of catecholamines in the blood. The mechanism by which this results in increased pulmonary vascular pressures is disputed. Factors probably include marked peripheral vasoconstriction, which shifts blood into the chest, acute left ventricular failure caused by profound systemic hypertension, or reduced compliance of the left ventricle resulting in the need for high filling pressures. However, what is not disputed is that pulmonary arterial wedge pressures are extremely high, and therefore of course the capillary pressures are high. It has also been shown that the oedema of neurogenic pulmonary oedema is of the high-permeability type, with elevated concentrations of high-molecular-weight proteins and cells.[8] Evidence therefore suggests that stress failure of pulmonary capillaries is involved. In addition, Minnear and colleagues[9,10] have shown that the changes in the lungs in experimental neurogenic pulmonary oedema are similar to those seen in rabbit lungs with stress failure.

High-altitude pulmonary oedema

High-altitude pulmonary oedema is probably something that many physicians never see. In California, high-altitude pulmonary oedema presents from time to time and it is certainly common in places like the Himalayas. It is known that there is a very strong association between the development of high-altitude pulmonary oedema and the degree of increase in pulmonary arterial pressure, as a result of hypoxic pulmonary vasoconstriction.[11] Interestingly, it has been shown a number of times that pulmonary artery wedge pressure is normal, suggesting that these patients do not have left ventricular failure. This is a high-permeability type of oedema with high concentrations of high-molecular-weight proteins and cells.[12] These concentrations are even higher than in acute respiratory distress syndrome (ARDS) which is thought of as the prime example of a high-permeability type of oedema. This is confusing since the mechanism of this type of oedema is presumed to be hydrostatic. It has been suggested that the hypoxic pulmonary vasoconstriction is uneven, and therefore those capillaries which are downstream from regions of constriction are protected from high pulmonary arterial pressure, but those capillaries that happened not to have a constricted region upstream of them will be damaged, due to exposure to the high pressure. In support of this, pathologists have described that foetal lung contains a very large amount of vascular smooth muscle but during the transition to adult life this vascular smooth muscle becomes involuted.[13]

Rats exposed to a low barometric pressure in a chamber develop disruptions of the blood-gas barrier, with escape of red blood cells from the capillary lumen into the interstitium and alveolar spaces.[14] These changes are consistent with ultrastructural findings in rabbits which develop capillary stress failure.[3] Another feature of high-altitude pulmonary oedema is that the bronchoalveolar lavage fluid contains high concentrations of leukotriene B_4 and other arachidonic acid metabolites, in addition to C5a complement fragments. This reflects similar findings in studies of rabbits with elevated transmural pressures. One source of the inflammatory mediators is likely to be alveolar macrophages which have become activated following exposure of the basement membranes as a result of disruption of the capillary endothelial cell layer.

Exercise-induced pulmonary haemorrhage

All thoroughbred racehorses in training show evidence of alveolar bleeding, with accumulation of haemosiderin-laden macrophages in their tracheal washings.[15] These animals have extremely high pulmonary vascular pressures. The left atrial pressure, measured with a catheter directly in the left atrium, is in the region of 70 mmHg,[16] due it is thought, to the extremely high filling pressures required by the right ventricle. The afterload of the left ventricular mean systemic pressure is 240 mmHg during racing and the pulmonary artery pressure 120 mmHg. However, pulmonary vascular resistance does not increase. The reason why the pulmonary artery pressure has risen is because the pulmonary venous pressure is so high. Even the pressure in the right atrium is 55 mmHg. These horses have been selectively bred to generate enormously high maximal oxygen consumption necessitating high cardiac outputs, and therefore extreme pulmonary vascular pressures.

Studies of the lungs of racehorses which have been exercised on a treadmill at high speed show that indeed there are breaks in the pulmonary capillaries.[17] However, it remains unclear as to how the phenomenon can be avoided since it appears to be an inevitable consequence of the extremely high vascular pressures which result from the very high aerobic activities. The finding in horses raises the question of whether elite human athletes also bleed into the alveoli, and haemoptysis has been reported anecdotally following severe exercise.[18] Subsequent studies showed that elite athletes do have some changes in their bronchial alveolar lavage fluid following extreme exercise. For example, the number of red blood cells in the bronchial alveolar lavage fluid was increased compared to sedentary controls and protein levels were higher. Athletes exercising at only 80% of the maximum oxygen consumption for an hour did not show similar abnormalities, except for increase in surfactant protein suggesting that it is only maximum exercise in elite athletes that causes the alterations in the blood-gas barrier.

Volume trauma

There have been numerous studies showing increased capillary permeability at high lung volumes, and it has also been shown that it is the high lung volumes that cause the damage to the capillaries, not the high pressure *per se*. It is important to note that it is volume trauma as opposed to barotrauma which causes these changes. This can be shown that by splinting the chest wall at the same alveolar pressure which prevents the high lung volume from occurring.[19] In rabbit studies when capillary transmural pressures are maintained, but lung volume is increased, it was found that there was a great increase in number of breaks both in the capillary endothelium and the alveolar epithelium.[20]

There is some evidence that the type of mechanical ventilation that is used affects the amount of capillary damage, particularly when patients are ventilated below the inflection point of a pressure–volume curve. The reason may be due to the distribution of stresses in the alveolar walls. In a normal lung, with normal alveolar mesh, where all the alveoli are the same size, the tension in the alveolar walls is uniform. However, if there is a region in the centre of the mesh which has a reduced alveolar volume, stresses in the immediate vicinity of this poorly expanded region are amplified. This may explain why patients ventilated below the inflection point on the pressure–volume curve, where there are areas of atelectasis in the lung, sustain more damage.

Structural failure of the capillary wall

Stress failure of the pulmonary capillaries may occur if the extracellular matrix is damaged. In Goodpasture's syndrome, autoantibodies attack the NC1 domain of type IV collagen, leading to weakening of the collagen and bleeding into the alveolar and glomerular spaces.[21]

Regulation of the structure of the blood-gas barrier

The blood-gas barrier presents a dilemma, brought about by the design requirements of the lung. It must be extremely thin to allow gas exchange by passive diffusion. However, at the same time integrity must be preserved when capillary pressure or lung volume rises. These are exacting requirements. If the blood-gas barrier is not thin enough there will be impairment of diffusion across the lung, seen for example in elite human athletes, where there is diffusion limitation of gas exchange, leading to a fall in arterial PO_2. It would clearly be advantageous in these circumstances to have a thinner blood-gas barrier, although this would predispose to alveolar oedema or haemorrhage or a combination of both. Again elite athletes apparently show a loss of integrity of the blood-gas barrier with increased numbers of red blood cells in the alveolar lavage fluid following maximal exercise.

It is possible that the capillary walls stretch, changing the wall stress and regulating the structure, particularly in terms of the amount of extracellular matrix type IV collagen in the alveolar walls. The alveolus may indeed sense more stress, regulating the structure of the wall, increasing or decreasing the amount of extracellular matrix proteins. Evidence that this may occur comes from observations in mitral stenosis. Typically, electron microscopy from patients with mitral stenosis show thickening of the basement membrane which is more pronounced in the capillary endothelial cell basement membrane than the basement membrane of the alveolar epithelial cell. This may suggest that the capillary endothelial cell deposits more collagen in response to stress. Mitral stenosis is a chronic condition but there is also the suggestion that similar regulation occurs over a shorter time span. In recent studies, anaesthetised open-chest rabbits had one lung ventilated with 8 cmH_2O of PEEP and the other lung ventilated at 1 cmH_2O of PEEP. Control rabbits were ventilated at 2 cmH_2O of PEEP in both lungs. In the animals that had one lung exposed to high levels of PEEP there was an increase in mRNA for pro-α-1 collagen, fibronectin and transforming growth factor-β1. These data suggest that the capillary wall components are continually being regulated in response to increased stress. In other studies of hypoxic animals, remodelling is rapid, with histological changes becoming evident after 2 days.[22,23] Excised pulmonary artery rings subjected to stretching expressed increased mRNA for pro-α-1 collagen within 4 hours in an endothelium-dependent process.[24]

Conclusion

In summary, the blood-gas barrier is an extremely vulnerable structure. The strength of the barrier can be attributed to an immensely thin layer of type IV collagen (50 nm) on the thin side of the blood-gas barrier. A number of pathological conditions occur due to stress failure of the pulmonary capillaries.

References

1 Gehr P, Bachofen M, Weibel ER. The normal human lung: ultrastructure and morphometric estimation of diffusion capacity. *Respir Physiol* 1978;**32**:121–40.
2 West JB, Tsukimoto K, Mathieu-Costello O, Prediletto R. Stress failure in pulmonary capillaries. *J Appl Physiol* 1991;**70**:1731–42.

3   Tsukimoto K, Mathieu-Costello O, Prediltto R, Elliott AR, West JB. *J Appl Physiol* 1991;**71**:573–82.

4   Yurchenco PD, Schittny JC. Molecular architecture of basement membranes. *FASEB J* 1990;**4**:1577–90.

5   Fein A, Grossman RF, Jones JG, Overland E, Pitts L, Murray JF, Staub NC. The value of edema fluid measurement in patients with pulmonary edema. *Am J Med* 1979;**67**:32–8.

6   Robin ED. Pulmonary edema. In: Fishman AP, Renkin EM, eds. *Pulmonary edema*. Bethesda, MD, American Physiological Society, 1979:217–28.

7   Sarnoff SJ, Berglund E, Sarnoff LC. Neurohemodynamics of pulmonary edema. *J Appl Physiol* 1981;**5**:367–74.

8   Cameron GR, De SN. Experimental pulmonary edema of nervous origin. *J Pathol Bacteriol* 1949;**61**:375–87.

9   Minnear FL, Connell RS. Increased permeability of the capillary–alveolar barriers in neurogenic pulmonary edema. *Microvasc Res* 1981;**22**:345–66.

10   Minnear FL, Kite C, Hill LA, Van Der Zee H. Endothelial injury and pulmonary congestion characterize neurogenic pulmonary edema in rabbits. *J Appl Physiol* 1987;**63**:335–41.

11   Hultgren HN, Grover RF, Hartley LH. Abnormal circulatory responses to high altitude in subjects with a previous history of high altitude pulmonary edema. *Circulation* 1997;**44**:759–70.

12   Hackett PH, Bertman J, Rodriguez G. Pulmonary edema fluid protein in high altitude pulmonary edema. *JAMA* 1986;**256**:36.

13   Reid L. The pulmonary circulation: remodelling in growth and disease. *Am Rev Respir Dis* 1979;**119**:531–46.

14   West JB, Colice GL, Lee Y-J *et al*. Pathogenesis of high altitude pulmonary oedema: direct evidence of stress failure of pulmonary capillaries. *Eur Respir J* 1995;**8**:523–9.

15   Whitwell KE, Greet TRC. Collection and evaluation of tracheobronchial washes in the horse. *Equine Vet* 1984;**16**:499–508.

16   Jones JH, Smith BL, Birks EK, Pascoe JR, Hughes TR. Left atrial and pulmonary artery pressures in exercising horses. *FASEB J* 1992;**6**:A2020 (abstract).

17   West JB, Mathieu-Costello O, Jones JH *et al*. Stress failure of pulmonary capillaries in racehorses with exercise induced pulmonary hemorrhage. *J Appl Physiol* 1993;**75L**:1097–9.

18   West JB, Mathieu-Costello O, Geddes DM. Intrapulmonary hemorrhage caused by stress failure of pulmonary capillaries during exercise. *Am Rev Respir Dis* 1991;**143**:A569 (abstract).

19   Hernandez LA, Peevy KJ, Moise AA, Parker JC. Chest wall restriction limits high airway pressure induced lung injury in young rabbits. *J Appl Physiol* 1989;**66**:2364–8.

20   Fu Z, Costello ML, Tsukimoto K *et al*. High lung volume increases stress failure in pulmonary capillaries. *J Appl Physiol* 1992;**73**:123–33.

21   Weislander J, Heinegard D. The involvement of type IV collagen in Goodpasture's syndrome. *Ann NY Acad Sci* 1985;**460**:363–74.

22   Meyrick B, Reid L. Hypoxia induced structural changes in the media and adventitia of the rat hilar pulmonary artery and their regression. *Am J Pathol* 1980;**100**:151–78.

23   Meyrick B, Reid L. The effect of continued hypoxia on rat pulmonary arterial circulation: an ultrastructural study. *Lab Invest* 1978;**38**:188–200.

24 Tozzi CA, Poiani GJ, Harangozo AM, Boyd CD, Riley DJ. Pressure induced connective tissue synthesis in pulmonary artery segments is dependent on intact endothelium. *J Clin Invest* 1989;**84**:1005–12.

25 Costello ML, Mathieu-Costello O, West JB. Stress failure of alveolar epithelial cells studied by scanning electron microscopy. *Am Rev Respir Dis* 1992;**145**:1446–55.

26 West JB, Mathieu-Costello O. Strength of the pulmonary blood-gas barrier. *Respir Physiol* 1992;**88**:141–8.

27 West JB, Mathieu-Costello O. Vulnerability of pulmonary capillaries in heart disease. *Circulation* 1995;**92**:622–31.